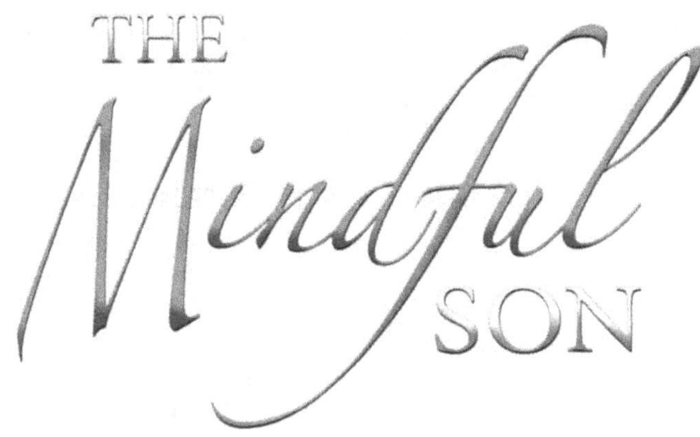

A Beacon of Hope Through the Storm of Mental Illness

Second Edition

James L. Hickman

Alpha Centauri Press
Hartselle, Alabama

2024 SECOND EDITION

ISBN: 978-0-9850856-3-6 | LCCN: 2024946789

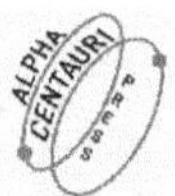

Alpha Centauri Press
603 Longhorn Pass, N.W., Suite 1B
Hartselle, AL 35640

MENTAL HEALTH PROFESSIONAL DISCLAIMER: This book does not and cannot contain mental health advice. The mental health information is provided for general informational and educational purposes only and is not a substitute for professional advice. Accordingly, before taking any actions based upon such information, we encourage you to consult with the appropriate professionals. We do not provide any kind of mental health advice. THE USE OR RELIANCE OF ANY INFORMATION CONTAINED IN THIS BOOK (OR EBOOK) OR RELATED WEBSITE(S) IS SOLELY AT YOUR OWN RISK.

Library of Congress Cataloging-in-Publication Data

Names: Hickman, James L., author

Title: The mindful Son: a beacon of hope through the storm of mental illness / James L. Hickman.

Description: Hartselle, Alabama: Alpha Centauri Press, [2024] | Summary: "James L. Hickman, licensed certified social worker, pens his autobiographical recounting which proves that recovery from serious mental illness is obtainable, while providing concrete information on how such recovery can be sustained." – Provided by publisher.

Identifiers: LCCN 2024946789 (print) Second Edition | ISBN: 978-0-9850856-3-6

Subjects: schizophrenia, mental illness, overcoming obstacles to quality mental health, suicide, post-psychotic depression, recovery from mental illness.

V10072024SC

Published in the United States of America

To consumers of mental health services the world over, their families, and the professionals who work hard for their betterment

ACKNOWLEDGMENTS

First, I want to thank the National Alliance on Mental Illness (NAMI) for the support this organization has provided me over the years. I want to express gratitude to all of the "NAMI Mommies," too many to list, who have encouraged me when I needed it most. Some of these beautiful ladies include Mary Reeder, Annita Thomas, Ann Denbo, Marilyn Volonino, Brenda Tanger, and Ethel Green.

I also want to thank Mike Autrey, now retired as the Director of the Office of Consumer Relations in Alabama, for supporting many of my endeavors. My friend and mentor, Walter Ballard, deserves recognition for inspiring and motivating me to be my best. Thomas Drinkard was immensely helpful in shaping the writing of this book through his work as my editor. Travis Tynan did a terrific job as my copy editor. Ellen Sallas helped me to make *The Mindful Son* available in e-book format. David Hitt was kind enough to write the foreword for this edition.

My brother, Albert Hickman, is an important part of my story, and I am grateful to him for being there. Tom, Dickie, and Petie Maynor, helped shape my life in many ways, throughout much of my story. Dickie Maynor has now gone to seek her heavenly reward, though she touched many lives with her grace, knowledge, and understanding. Heather Jacoby, may she rest in peace, was my best friend and companion for many years following the completion of the first edition, and she is sorely missed.

Marilyn Lands and Bernice Maze, now retired from the profession of psychotherapy, helped save my life through their work. Faye Porter and Ann Murray, also retired from mental health service, were also influential in my recovery story. Reverend Curtis Thomas, who entered eternal glory, advised me in spiritual matters during the completion of this book. All praise and honor for this project ultimately go to God, whom I thank continuously for allowing me to be its steward.

List of Abbreviations

AAMU: Alabama Agricultural and Mechanical University

CMHS: Consumers of Mental Health Services

CRDC: Consumer Run Drop-in Center

DMCC: Decatur Morgan Counseling Center

DHR: Department of Human Resources

HMCMHC: Huntsville/Madison County Mental Health Center

LSAT: Law School Admission Test

MHA: Mental Health Association

MHCNCA: Mental Health Center of North Central Alabama

MSW: Master's Degree in Social Work

NAMI: National Alliance for Mental Illness

NARH: North Alabama Regional Hospital

NASA: National Aeronautics and Space Administration

PLA: People Living with Addictions

PLMI: People Living with Mental Illness

SMI: Serious Mental Illness

SSA: Social Security Administration

UA: University of Alabama

UAH: University of Alabama in Huntsville

UASL: University of Alabama School of Law

UHC: University Health Center

VRS: Vocational Rehabilitation Services

TABLE OF CONTENTS

FOREWORD

It would be all-too-cliché for a foreword to call the book it is introducing "life-changing."

Without doubt, there lies between its covers that sort of potential. For some readers, it hopefully will be. For others, it will "merely" be a powerful story that offers renewed empathy for those around them.

I was honored when Jim asked me to write the foreword for this second edition of *The Mindful Son*.

To the best of my knowledge, Jim and I are the only two published authors to come from the graduating Class of 1992 of Huntsville High School in Alabama's Rocket City. My own books, *Homesteading Space* and *Bold They Rise*, are appropriate fare for a city that once billed itself as The Space Capital of the World – the stories of the Skylab program (co-written with two astronauts who lived aboard that space station) and the early years of the Space Shuttle Program. It's not unusual for me to be asked to read a manuscript or offer a blurb for books about space. Writing a foreword for a book on mental health? This was a first for me. But it was an invitation I accepted eagerly, and I am privileged to undertake.

Confession time – when I heard that Jim had published a book, I went out immediately and bought a copy. And, just as immediately, didn't read it. I thought from the title I knew what it was. I put it on the shelf of books I fully intend to get to before too long, and it sat there, honestly, for years before I finally picked it up. I was wrong about what I thought it was.

The same, I should note, I now know is also true for Jim. From the time my family moved back to Huntsville halfway through sixth grade, we were in classes together. Sharing the first two letters of our last names meant we were often in homeroom together. We were friends, but in a "person I like at school" way, not a "hanging out at each other's house" way. That's far less a reflection of him or our friendship than on me – I don't know that a handful of my classmates were ever in my home. But as a result, while I knew Jim, I only knew the at-school Jim. Reading this book, learning about his home life in those years, introduced me to a Jim I never knew at all.

I share all that because, for me, it was a huge part of the moral of this story. You can know someone, and utterly not know someone, all at once. You can see the cover, but not know the book.

What do our books have in common? We both share explorations of alien worlds. If you've never lived in space, the only way you can understand it is to hear about it from someone who has. You can know the facts, but they're not the reality. You could know how to do the math to calculate the orbital mechanics of keeping a spaceship in zero-g circling Earth and still have no clue *what it's like* to float around like Superman or stare down at our beautiful blue planet with a God's-eye view. You can be informed with a wealth of data about mental illness and yet have no clue what it's like to be a person living with it.

Like nothing I have read, *The Mindful Son* shares that experience. Not the facts and the data and diagnoses and the indications, but the *what it's like.* He throws open the curtains and lets the world in, in a way that is incredibly vulnerable and incredibly brave and incredibly powerful.

Powerful enough to change a life.

Powerful, for those with a loved one living with mental illness, in its ability to help the reader understand. Jim walks the reader through his dark times living with schizophrenia in a remarkably matter-of-fact manner. An outsider might see his thoughts during those times as madness, but to the one living them, they were divinest sense. And that is how he recounts them, unapologetically and unvarnished, in a way I've not seen before. There is life-changing power here to help that reader understand and support that loved one in a way they currently cannot.

Powerful, for those living with mental illness, for its story of hope. This is a story of a descent into darkness, but it's also a story of a return to light, sharing a road to recovery that doubles as a roadmap. This second edition conveys that even more powerfully – the book does not have a "happy ending," because that would mean Jim's story had ended, but seeing the story years further down the road shows the tenacity of its hope. There is life-changing power here in its delivery of hope to a situation that has deep momentum toward hopelessness.

And so, this book may not change your life. Some readers may not need to hear its message, or may have already received it. If that's you, I hope you find this a fascinating and compelling read that captivates you with its unique perspective.

But, for those who need it, I hope this book finds its way to you. And I hope it changes your life.

David Hitt

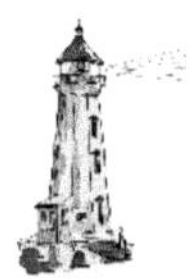

PROLOGUE

The writers of fiction say that it feels to them as if the story they are telling is truly occurring, perhaps on some distant plane of reality. Although, my account really happened in this existence, the memories I invoke to assemble this memoir seem strangely surreal. I don't know if my mind contains some work of fiction within its depths, and I am unlikely to ever find out until I share my story of real-life wonder with you.

How many fiction writers, who feel in some dark corner of their imagination that their stories may actually be real in some far-off place, would continue writing if they were suddenly characters in their own works? Would a seer of such realities continue to write if he knew he stood a good chance of being roasted by a dragon or framed for some crime he had not committed?

As the chronicler of my own journey of recovery from serious mental illness, I can't afford to dwell long on such questions.

While I assure you that I will not reveal to you at the end of the story that it is all a dream, I cannot promise you that aspects of it will not seem like one.

At age seven, I lost my mother to schizophrenia when she passed away unexpectedly. Thanks to the loving care of my maternal grandmother, among others, by the time I was twenty-one I was primed to enter law school. That same year, I too was diagnosed with this devastating disorder following my first psychotic break from reality.

The year before I was diagnosed with my illness, I pedaled a bicycle across the country to raise money for children with disabilities. I never suspected that I would soon have a disability of my own.

I was eventually in a position to remain in recovery from

schizophrenia, and to provide care for other people living with mental illness as a health care professional. Ultimately, I was able to rescue my older brother, Bert, also diagnosed with schizophrenia, from homelessness.

I have known vexing poverty and ample surplus in successive waves. I have been friendless and I have been loved by all. I have known hunger as an orphan without an attentive parent and been spoiled with advantages few can claim. I have been considered a fool and a genius, depending upon when people crossed my path. I have been a slacker and an athletic champion, depending upon my frame of mind. A failure and a success: I finally learned what it takes to remain on top.

The events described in this journey you are embarking upon with me are significant for a variety of reasons. Anyone who seeks an understanding of what having a mental illness is, will discover it these pages. They prove beyond doubt that recovery from serious mental illness is attainable, and they provide concrete information on how this recovery can be sustained.

The wisdom I acquired through years of trial and error is now at the disposal of anyone who reads these words.

This story is inspirational! Anyone who reads this book will know that great obstacles are surmountable with determination and the application of certain principles.

Greater understanding of the community of people with mental illness and their families will be fostered in my account. Professional providers of mental health care are special people, and this book is a window into their world as well.

This is the story of the ultimate triumph of a family devastated by mental illness over the course of thirty-four years. Many dark days are recounted in this voyage, until we finally reach the light together.

I have become a messenger of good omen, though its delivery is arduous and has left indelible marks upon my spirit. It is with a free heart that I now proclaim its contents to you.

REFLECTIONS

It is the summer of 1995 and I am pedaling an Italian road bicycle across the Texas plain. The thin tires are reinforced with a special tape to support the chubby body with which I began this journey, a month ago. Thirty pounds of my flesh has now been scoured and melted away by relentless exercise in the summer sun. I, along with one-hundred of my fraternity brothers from across the nation have chosen to spend our summer making this trek in order to raise money for children with disabilities.

I am an American Studies Major at the University of Alabama (UA), home of the Crimson Tide, and this trip seems to fit perfectly with my chosen field of study. In American Studies I have learned a great deal about the history, sociology, and literary tradition of the nation. Now I am examining much of its topography in a very personal way as I watch my sweat drip to the earth for mile after punishing mile.

The Crimson Tide won the national championship in football in 1992, my freshman year. I was a football champion on a city level in my hometown of Huntsville, Alabama, but three years and too many keg parties to count have taken place since I wore a pair of cleats.

The cleats I now wear are fitted to the pedals of my bicycle. Their special design locks into place with a twist of my ankles. I had no idea that these shoes were a vital part of the gear I would need for my trip until I had already pedaled halfway across California. It was then that the reality of what I had gotten myself into really clicked in my mind. I was considered a Fitness Champion at Huntsville High School, and had my picture taken for the yearbook.

Three years is certainly a long time to refrain from any form of physical exercise. This really dawned upon me the first day of our journey, when we crossed The Golden Gate Bridge in San Francisco. Mark Twain always said that the coldest winter he ever spent was a summer in San Francisco. Now I know what he meant.

The third day of our trip, I was told that we would be climbing the Sierra Nevada Mountains. Pushing that bicycle by hand up a mountain was a challenge. But when it started snowing on us, the task became that much more demanding. Who would have thought that snow could fall in such soul aching drifts—and in the middle of June? When one of our support vans finally rolled up beside me to carry me the rest of the way up the mountain, I didn't protest.

Rolled up in the blankets in the ski lodge at the top of the mountain, I still couldn't shake that cold from my bones. The next day, the vans had to shuttle all of us down the other side of the mountain to Carson City, Nevada, the state's capitol. Our leaders informed us that bicycling downhill on ice at those speeds posed too much of a risk to our safety. I had no problem with their assessment as the idea of being splattered all over the side of a mountain would not be an appealing idea, neither to me nor the grandmother who raised me.

I want to attend the University of Alabama, School of Law (UASL) after I graduate next year. I worked there as a copier's assistant all last year and have labored persistently to maintain a high grade point average. The UASL is extremely competitive, after all, and it will take more than the relationships I have cultivated with many of the law professors to pave my way there.

For now, I must pedal along this dreary highway, foot after foot, mile after mile. But at least I am in great shape again, and the journey is not as grueling as when I first began. Since I began this tour, I have slept beneath a blanket of desert stars and camped by a murmuring river at the bottom of a canyon inhabited by Native Americans. I have gotten in closer touch with my dreams, and each mile I complete I know will bring me closer to seeing them coalesce into a beautiful reality.

A semi-truck is hurtling past me. A rock spins off one of its tires and bounces off of my helmeted head. Another one strikes me in the abdomen a microsecond later, and I feel the sharp pain throb in my gut. A feeling of despair washes over me as I contemplate how much more of this trip

I have to endure. I pedal harder now, resolved to continue on, thankful that one of the rocks didn't knock my teeth out. My mind begins to wander further now into the depths of my past, visualizing some of the obstacles I have already faced.

I was born in 1974, and by 1975 my mother had been diagnosed with schizophrenia, one of the world's most devastating mental illnesses. It often strikes women following childbirth. When it struck my mother, far less than now was known about how to treat this illness, and the medication available in those years was not nearly as effective as today's.

The disease coursed ferociously through my mother's mind and she was never the same again. She constantly suffered frightening hallucinations and delusions, and was drained of energy by the disease and the myriad of medications she was now forced to swallow. My mother and father were divorced shortly after her diagnosis.

At age two I was removed from the custody of my mother by the court, on the recommendation of the Alabama Department of Human Resources. I lived in a series of foster homes until age four, when I moved with my father and older brother to Portland, Oregon.

For our first year there, my brother and I lived in relative comfort, living with a stepmother and three stepsisters who ranged in age from twelve to eighteen. We lived in a suburban environment which was entirely new and different from the rural environment I was accustomed to. Riding my big wheel through the suburban streets filled with other children and houses was a pleasure. I also saw my first movie in a movie theater (The Muppet Movie) and rode an escalator in a new place I discovered called a mall.

In the second year of our life in Oregon, though, my father and my stepmother divorced, and Bert and I moved into an apartment complex with our father in a poorer neighborhood. During those formative years, my primal instincts were activated as I confronted poverty, hunger, and neglect. I learned to navigate the world of older and larger children who were also impoverished but who at least all seemed to have parents who were present in their lives. My father drank heavily and would leave my brother Bert and me to fend for ourselves for weeks at a time.

After my mother had been married to my stepfather, Dave, for a time, the Alabama Department of Human Resources urged the court to return custody of Bert and me back to my mother. By the time we moved back to Alabama with my mother and stepfather, both of us had been altered emotionally by our experiences in Oregon, much the way our mother had been altered by her mental illness. Her appearance was usually somewhat disheveled, and she often had a look on her face as if her mind was in some place far distant from where her body was.

Living with my mother, I saw her affected by the symptoms of her illness in other ways. On one occasion, she hailed down a passing police car and swore to them that somebody was out to cause harm to herself and her children. Then she disappeared for a time and I was told that she was in the hospital. This was a recurring theme of all the delusions I saw her struggle with in my short time with her.

After a year of living with my mother, she passed away. I never learned exactly what the circumstances of her death were. I was simply told that she had a heart attack. When Dave informed my grandmother and me what had happened, I went out to the dogwood tree in my grandmother's yard and just sat there, feeling numb inside.

From then on, I was reared primarily by my grandmother, Colice, who was assisted by a hodgepodge of families. Dave continued to support my family financially, and emotionally. My brother Bert continued to live in Dave's home until he was twenty-five. Dave was a highly intelligent engineer, and he did much to ensure that his stepchildren developed an intellectual mindset. He always wore threadbare clothes that he had purchased from the Goodwill store that made him look very much like a Caucasian-looking version of Gandhi.

My grandmother had formerly been a wealthy businesswoman. However, she had spent vast sums of money in her attempt to maintain the well-being of my mother. She often wore once-expensive pant suits that had become somewhat outdated, and tended to give her the regal mystique of a Buddha.

What remained of her fortune was a duplex house in a working-class neighborhood. When I was ten years old, Grandmother sold the duplex and moved us to an apartment complex in a wealthier part of Huntsville. From then on, I attended those schools that my grandmother considered the finest in our community. I eventually became the third generation of my family to graduate from Huntsville High School and had the opportunity—thanks to my grandmother, stepfather, and federal Pell grants—to attend the UA.

The events of my childhood are far more complex than can be summed up in a few words, and are certain to be of interest to people. Experts in mental health matters, of all persuasions, will want to understand the full nature of my childhood in their attempt to understand the man who appeared to face the daunting obstacle of serious mental illness.

I'm back on my bicycle again. This time I'm pedaling from east to west across my home state of Alabama. I am very excited about our destination for today, which is the Omicron Chapter of the Pi Kappa Phi fraternity. The old fraternity house lies on the campus of the UA, and is the place where I have lived, excluding summers, for the past two years. The Journey of Hope won't end until we reach Charleston, South Carolina, but reaching my home campus will mark a special milestone for me. I can't wait to see the reactions of the fraternity brothers of my home chapter when they see that I have really made it this far. Today, my excitement about traveling to the ultimate symbol of the end to this intense odyssey propels me to the head of the line of cyclists.

I find myself pedaling faster than I ever have before, as I feel my strong, new-found muscles pushing my body into a higher gear. I had no idea that I was capable of riding this fast and am elated to see that I am managing to maintain my lead. This is not a race, and every day up until now, I have been content to be one of the last riders to make it in each day. My group of riders tends to be the most pessimistic about our journey, as well as the ones most eager to reach our final destination. We are affectionately termed by the other cyclists as the Delta Lambdas, for the Greek letters D and L, which stand for Dead Last.

As we reach the ending point of today's ride, one of the riders from the state of Washington is following right behind me, smiling as he encourages me forward. For that brief moment in time, I feel the sense of gloom which has hovered around me throughout my journey vanish, and now I only see the victory at hand.

I am proving to my friends and family, who thought this journey sounded impossible, that I can do whatever I set my mind to. I am not thinking about the many obstacles I have traversed to reach this point, and I am entirely unaware of the mountains of despair I will face in my near future. For this one sunny afternoon of pure joy, I am aware only of the feeling of elation as I cross the finish line, home.

THE UNRAVELING

During the summer of 1996, I gazed at a bright-eyed woman in an English class at the University of Alabama, Tuscaloosa. As class ended for the day, we began a conversation. Our dialogue was perfection; I felt that I could almost hear in my mind what she was about to say before she uttered each word.

Why shouldn't I hear what she said before she vocalized it? Hadn't my friend Tommy, just the other day, confessed to me that he thought that we could evolve to a point where it was possible to read minds? It was that simple. Fantasy and reality merged in a way to alter the path of my faculties. I danced out of the old school building, giddy about my love connection, as well as my newly discovered power of telepathy.

As I walked to my car across campus to make the drive home, I discovered that I was not just catching a stray thought from the woman I was wooing, but also hearing the thoughts of anyone who crossed my path. My mental abilities were also augmented by a phenomenon in which I began deriving meanings from every idea that seemed to be related to anything else, based on the thinnest thread of evidence. Anyone who glanced my way was doing so because they, too, could read minds. I was sinking into the world of the supernatural which contained forces which were, at first, subtle, but were inexorably sucking me into a dark whirlpool. Ideas began to blend as I would think of one concept and would soon be linking it with another at such a rate that it was impossible to understand what anybody was really saying.

The class I'd been attending when the phenomenon first appeared was based on Twin Peaks, a television show perfectly designed to have no real meaning. Trying to make sense of the show's loose connection of plots and themes only bolstered my state of confusion. I did well in the class for another week, but then found myself completely unable to concentrate on anything as my brain overextended its abilities, trying to keep up with the rapid pace of sensory input.

One week following this initial chaos, I was lying on a hammock while Tommy was visiting me at the house I had recently moved into. I tried to describe to him how my mind was buzzing as I glared into the blue ether of sky.

"I feel like I'm really zoning out, and I can't think clearly at all."

"I think you should try to take it easy," was his reply.

Unbeknownst to us, a serious mental disorder had crept into my life and was beginning to take root. It seems almost strange in hindsight that the concept that I was experiencing some mental aberration never occurred to me. I thought I was experiencing some sort of awakening in my mind, wherein I was gaining incredible mental abilities. I believed that this transformation was leaving me temporarily debilitated, until I completed this metamorphosis. This notion was exciting as I contemplated my newfound abilities. Exhilaration abruptly became terror when I made a telephone call to my grandmother a couple of days later.

I was in perfect cheer as I described to her my experience of finishing college, failing to mention that I had now become telepathic. At the end of the conversation she laughed loudly at something I said, and in my mind I could hear the laughter amplified, as if someone else were laughing inside my mind. A state of confusion superseded my elated state of mind as I hung up the phone. After careful contemplation of the situation, it seemed that one of my English professors, a man in late middle age, had been the one laughing in my head in unison with my grandmother.

Incredible! Somehow, my grandmother had known about the awakening of my new powers the whole time. My professor also had this strange mental gift of telepathy and he noticed me in his class as someone who had the potential to read minds. These strange theories bombarded me throughout the evening and as I prepared to fall asleep that night. I was sure that my professor and my grandmother were forming some sort of union, with me as the catalyst. They even began carrying on whole conversations in my mind. They said that they were like psychic vampires and I was going along for the ride. I eventually fell asleep as the conversation continued, independent of my awareness.

I awoke at four o'clock in the morning and was conscious for only an instant before I realized, with dawning horror, what I thought had occurred. All of the religion I had largely abandoned in my college years came rushing back instantly, and I felt guilty of an enormous moral crime. The thought that I had agreed to merge with vampires left me fearing for my mortal soul, as I remembered that this was something contrary to God's will. My roommate was an avid hunter, and a mounted deer's head, bristling with massive antlers, stared at me from the wall opposite my bed. Suddenly, I could see in the darkness of my room that the animal's eyes glowed! The blue luminescence of the animal's stare gripped my heart in terror!

I turned on the light switch, grabbing for the nine millimeter pistol I kept underneath my bed. I thought that my roommate was one of the vampires and would burst into my room with one of his hunting rifles at any moment. Gangster rap songs pulsed through my brain as I prepared myself to face the monstrous attack.

After an hour of preparing for the feared ambush, I heard other Voices begin to speak inside my mind. These Voices were telling me to put the pistol down; that the only way to get myself out of this mess was to beg God's forgiveness and do what they said. The Voices seemed like a combination of many of my professors, other than the one I thought was a vampire. They were robed in white, and they were saying that they were an academy of good, and that they wanted me to be a new member. I said that I would listen to them, and I pleaded with God to forgive me for allowing the union between my grandmother and my English professor, which my mind was convinced had taken place. The Voices told me to leave the house instantly, without a weapon. I packed my clothes and my possessions, including my gun, in two laundry baskets and headed for my old car. I placed the baskets on top of the car and the Voices told me to leave them there. I entered the car and drove off, allowing all of my possessions to spill out on to the street.

The Voices then told me to drive straight ahead. In a couple of minutes, I entered Tuscaloosa's small downtown area going about thirty five miles per hour. At the traffic lights, the Voices told me to drive through them with my eyes closed, and I followed their instructions, zooming through the intersection unscathed. Eventually, I reached the end of the street and parked the car there. I began walking aimlessly around town and had completely lost track of where I'd abandoned the car. I walked around all that day, thinking about the bizarre occurrences that I had been witness to. No matter how hard I thought about it all, I couldn't understand how all of the supernatural pieces fit together. After a time, I found myself on the campus and noticed a green knoll watered by a sprinkler system. The good Voices, who wanted me to be redeemed from the unholy happenings of the previous night, told me in angelic tones to kneel down there.

As the sprinkler water showered me with droplets of cold pain, I felt something vile inside me being destroyed. I continued my wandering, and at about midday I called my grandmother from a pay telephone. I no longer felt that she and the professor were really a part of the hostile takeover of my soul. I told her I was walking around in the sun, that I could not find my car, and that I was very confused. Even then, I felt the irony. My grandmother had dealt with similar situations involving my mother. The fact that she was now forced to relive a comparable situation caused me to tremble with shame and guilt. While I could see the similarities in the condition of my mother and in what I seemed to be experiencing, I did not believe that I was exhibiting symptoms of mental illness. The bizarre events that had unfolded seemed quite real, even though I had not quite yet made sense of how they affected me.

I managed to find my way to my friend Tommy's house by evening. I didn't tell him many details, but I explained to him that I was zoning out badly and had managed to lose my car. He drove me around and, to my relief, helped me locate it.

When we got back to his place, he took me to a darkly lighted room decorated in a psychedelic manner, with fluorescent artwork and designs. We had a long discussion that wound up being theological in nature. I had lost much of my faith around my sophomore year and had become an agnostic. Tommy talked about how no matter how many powerful entities in the universe might exist, that there was one all-powerful and benevolent force that was more prevailing than them all, and that was God.

The conversation was very helpful to me in terms of gaining some perspective about what I was experiencing, and it added passion to my decision to believe in God once again. We ate Chinese food and watched Star Trek as my mind relaxed a bit, and he talked me into going back to my roommate's house. When I arrived there, my roommate was happy to see me and concerned about finding my things out in the middle of the street. I then realized with quickening horror that my gun had been among the items that fell out, and that it was now missing. My worry magnified as I realized that there was an elementary school right next door to the house. I could envision a child finding the gun, picking it up, and doing heaven knows what with it. I had my friend drive me down to the police station, and I explained to the officers that I had lost the gun and where I had lost it, even though I did not have a satisfactory explanation for how it had disappeared. A police report was typed out but I was asked no further questions.

For the next three days, I quit eating, as my body simply stopped letting me know that it required food, and I ceased going to classes. I had been hired that summer to work at the UASL. However, I hadn't showed up to work for a week since I began hearing the Voices. When I finally returned to the UASL, it was not to work, but to investigate the supernatural phenomenon I had been experiencing. I completely avoided my boss, who was in the copy room downstairs, in order to reach my new objective. I went straight up the Lego block stairs of the art deco building to talk to one of the law professors I knew. He had been my teacher in an undergraduate constitutional history class. He had been one of the spiritual gurus speaking in my mind, and I thought he had answers for me. I walked into his office, and I asked him something about his experience in the Vietnam War, and referred to the fact that I had seen visions and experienced some supernatural phenomenon.

"Can you help me figure out what is going on?" I asked. "No I can't, but I suggest you go to the University Health Center," was his curt reply.

I loped away from the UASL, feeling disappointed and not really thinking that the University Health Center (UHC) held any answers for me. My professor's manner did plant a seed in my mind that what was occurring to me could be related, in some way, to mental illness. I was not yet willing, though, to accept that possibility as a realistic answer to what I was experiencing. I walked past the UHC and to the office of the professor who I originally thought had invaded my mind, along with my grandmother. Maybe he could explain to me what was actually going on, or what I should do next. I entered his dark office located in a building that looked like a parapet of a castle, thankful to find that he was there. I first mentioned to him that I believed his daughter, who was in my Twin Peaks class, was dating the man teaching the class. This I had concocted from all of the symbolism and linking of themes that had been flying around the classroom.

"That is not the case, at all. I don't know what you're talking about, young man," he said.

Holding up my index finger to him and feeling the magic of what it symbolized, I told him that I had concluded that there was one God and that his goodness would always prevail over any kind of evil.

"God revealed all of this to me, you see. You have to understand that he keeps showing me signs of all manner of things," I explained.

He had a stunned, fearful look on his face as I spoke.

"I'm running late for a meeting," he said.

His steps down the stairs were long and quick to get away from me. I followed him for a way across the campus wishing he would reveal something more.

He then turned back to me and said very sternly, "Don't do anything stupid!"

I decided then to start walking in the direction of my old fraternity house. His strides lengthened as he put space between us.

Punching the secret code into the door lock of my old fraternity house, I quickly made my way to my former room. A month earlier, I had bidden farewell to the aged mansion. I'd never expected to lay my head down in there again. The colonial style house, closed for the summer, had no electricity. Even so, I still felt comfortable in the isolation of the small room where I'd lived for the past three years, except for summers. My consolation would be short lived. As I lay on the bare mattress on the floor, I began to sense the presence of great evil that lived in the old house. The fraternal rituals I had participated in over the years rushed back to my mind in an alarming way. I imagined the hooded spirits who wanted to destroy my soul stalking down the hallways outside my door. They were brandishing ceremonial knives and daring me to leave the confines of my little room. I felt protected, somehow, in my little cell where I had worked so diligently on my studies through the years. I managed to fall asleep in the abandoned house, despite the nocturnal spirits looming.

The next morning, I found a black covered notebook with some of my scribbling from one of my classes in my closet and began what I believed to be the final test. In the middle of the notebook, which had suddenly gained profound significance for me, I wrote in large letters the word God and circled it. I left the notebook on my old mattress, not really knowing who, if anybody would find it. I fled from the once again abandoned dwelling and began my journey on foot. It was raining heavily, and as I passed the ancient trees on the campus, I saw that lightning had splintered one. The angelic Voices, which had guided me so clearly earlier on, told me I would not need my watch. I took off my plastic digital and added it to the rain drops dappling a puddle of water, never breaking stride.

I walked on past the campus and became hopelessly lost in the twists and turns of the surrounding town. As the rain stopped, I came to an old storefront and saw a solitary wooden chair. One of the Voices that was neither male nor female, but seemed to be comprised of pure thought energy, told me to sit there. I sat there for perhaps an hour or two before an older man asked me what I was doing. I told him I was just sitting there, and a police car arrived soon after. The police officer told me I should keep moving, and so I did. I walked on into isolated neighborhoods that were more densely surrounded by trees, vines, and other vegetation I was not familiar with. This area was more untamed than the garden-like confines of the campus.

A Voice that sounded like God commanded me not to eat anything and to just drink water. I managed to drink a glass of water or two at a tiny restaurant, hidden by trees and isolated from anything else even remotely resembling a business. I was really becoming dehydrated as I made my long journey. I had not eaten a morsel of food in many days and my mind and body felt weakened by this fast, as well as my surreal experiences.

I hitched a ride for a short distance with an older man who was driving an old car, but I did not really know where I was going.

When it finally dawned on the man that I had no physical destination, he said, “Well, I guess I’d better let you off here.”

As I walked down strange roads, I thought of Jesus, Buddha, and all of the holy people throughout history. I thought that perhaps I was chosen as a messiah to be sent to another world. In truth, there were so many theories streaming through my mind that it is impossible to remember them all.

At one point, after it resumed raining, one of my fraternity brothers was driving by and happened to spot me. He called out to me. I said nothing. The Commanding Voice of God told me not to talk to him. He drove slowly for five minutes or so trying to talk me into getting into the car, but the Voice insisted that he was not a part of my journey. Eventually, he drove away.

After another couple of hours of walking, I made it to an area that was wooded and crosshatched by a maze of trails and gravel paths that left me completely lost. After wandering for a short time, I realized that I had actually been here once before. My roommate had driven me out there in his truck one day to show me some of his grandfather's land, and I could see what appeared to be the same small oil wells dotting the landscape. Images of vampires and werewolves sprang suddenly to mind so that each path appeared foreboding.

I walked around in circles trying to escape the place, but everywhere I turned, there were more darkening woods. It was now twilight, and at this point I was frantic to find my way out of there. I did not want to be stuck out there at night, at the mercy of the place's nighttime denizens. I came to a stream and God's Voice said I should swim in it.

I slipped first my body and then my head into the murky, chest deep, water and felt refreshed by its welcoming pull. As thirsty as I was, I could not help but gulp several mouthfuls of the silt liquid. With my thirst somewhat slaked, I began to float down the stream, allowing my senses to soak in the primeval woods and water. As I continued to drift down the stream, allowing the water to course through my system, it felt as if the animal part of my being was somehow being drawn out of the intangible spiritual aspect of my self.

For a moment, I felt as if I were some sort of reptile returning to the primordial realm, which my ancestors had left behind millennia before. After about five minutes of floating, I left the stream and headed for the thicket of trees and brush on the right-hand bank. I crawled my way through the tangled tunnel of growth until I came to a gravel path, bordered by trees marked with orange tape. These, too, I had seen on my previous trip to these woods.

I prayed to God, asking him to show me the way, and after several correctly taken turns I was thankful to find myself on a standard paved road. Elated, I walked down the road surrounded by even more trees until I came to an intersection. I prayed to God, asking him to help me to make the correct choice again. I turned right and walked down the road for a few minutes before I was pleased to see a small church in the distance. Surely, I would find refuge there. I quickened my pace, though my feet were aching and waterlogged. When I arrived at the tiny, whitewashed building, I found it locked and closed for the day; but still, a sense of serenity settled on me in the presence of this sacred shrine. I sat on the smoothly polished concrete entrance, thinking about the old-time sermons that must certainly be held there, replete with a minister who wore slicked back hair. I was so thirsty I tried to rub the residue of a small puddle for its moisture to place it on my tongue. I was very tired and wanted my journey to end, but after God's Voice told me I must continue I resumed my trek down the road.

The light faded into dusk as I came upon a row of distantly spaced one-story houses. God's Voice told me to ask for the things I needed from the people along the path. I stopped at a brick house and knocked on the door. After my encounter with the river and dense forest, I'm sure I must have been an unwelcome sight. A man in his thirties wearing a ball cap answered the door and I asked him for some water. He returned handing me a plastic bottle of cold water. I thanked him for it as I twisted off the cap. In no time, I felt its cooling contents trickle down my throat.

"This idea seems to be working," I said to myself, as I continued down the row of widely spaced houses.

By this time, the country road had completely darkened into night. I decided to go to another house, and when an older looking man, who seemed vaguely ex-military, answered the door, I asked him, "Do you have a bed where I might sleep for the night?"

"No, I don't," he said, slamming the door closed.

I resumed walking down the darkened road, and after about ten minutes had passed, a police car pulled up next to me with the older man I had just spoken to in the passenger seat, glaring at me as if he had been deputized. The police officer driving the car asked me if I had a place to stay.

"I don't have anywhere to go," I said curtly.

He ushered me into the back of the police car and asked where he should take me.

"Just take me to the homeless shelter," I said, realizing that finding someone to take me into his or her home was not to be part of my journey.

"Don't you want to go to the hospital?" the older man asked.

I had not made this journey simply to end it now.

"The homeless shelter will be fine, thank you," I replied.

Grudgingly, they dropped me off at a small shelter in a rural setting. I was greeted by a middle-aged black attendant, who did not quite seem to know what to make of me. After filling out a questionnaire asking me some basic information, like my name, height, and weight, I was ushered into a room with two rows of bunk beds and given an upper cot.

The ragged men milling about the bunk beds really frightened me, in my state of mind, though they all kept a silent distance from me. I woke up in the middle of the night with visions of demon-possessed men molesting me in some manner. Early in the morning, without saying a word to anyone, I fled the shelter and its occupants. The sun had just risen and the sky looked stunningly beautiful, as the world seemed to stand still. I walked down the street having absolutely no idea where I was.

I imagined myself on a hill above the university preaching to the masses. I walked about a quarter of a mile or so contemplating this idea when I passed a convenience store, which was closed, just like everything else in this new world. There was a poster on the window that illustrated a soul singer whose first name was Marvin. My mind quickly associated this image with Marvin the houseman who worked in our fraternity house.

Marvin was a middle-aged black man who had worked at the old house for decades doing minor jobs, and he was the target of much jest and many practical jokes. I spoke to him on many occasions and seemed to do so more often than any of the other fraternity brothers.

The man I was now seeing in the poster was somehow Marvin the houseman's alter ego. The soul singer moaning painfully into the microphone looked as if he was privy to some ancient mystery. Yes, it all made sense! Marvin somehow thrived on the debauchery enacted by the unknowing college students. He was a psychic vampire, or perhaps a demon.

I walked a little further and came across some sort of small manufacturing plant. The place projected an abysmal aura, as if it were a whirlpool sucking in human misery. When I walked into the darkened corridors of the place, I thought I had entered the mechanized bowels of hell. A grizzled woman pointed to a ledger and told me to sign it as if I belonged there. I beat a hasty retreat in the opposite direction of the woman to a gazebo that sat outside the tiny factory. God's Voice commanded me to sit down and keep my eyes closed and not to say anything. Shaking with fear, I did as I was told.

Soon, I was overhearing a conversation made by what sounded to me like a black man who was talking to somebody on a telephone. He was arguing profanely with someone about the custody of a child. From what I understood, the child had a white mother.

I interpreted this conversation to mean that the man was the devil arguing over my fate. That conversation died away and I was then hearing voices of people sitting around me in the gazebo, engaging in casual conversation. Eventually it died away and I continued to focus on keeping my eyes closed like God's Voice had told me to. Eventually, I could not resist opening my eyes for a quick peak, and what I saw startled me. I saw a black man, about my age, sitting directly across from me. He was looking back at me and seemed to be mimicking my facial expressions. It was like a mirror reflection of me, if I were black instead of white. I closed my eyes again and kept them closed. Was everything I had been experiencing somehow about race?

I had spent a great deal of time learning about racial issues in my American Studies classes, which focused heavily on the contributions and history of ethnic minorities. I had no idea then that in the future I would have the opportunity to learn far more about these issues. At that time, all I could think was, "Lord what should I do next?"

I heard God's Voice telling me to get up and walk away, keeping my eyes shut, as I did so. After a time, he told me that I could open my eyes, and as I did I saw an eighteen-wheeler whizzing by. I walked down the road until I saw a convenience store. I continued wandering toward it. An elderly black man, dressed in farmer's clothes came out of the store. I asked him if he would give me a ride, thinking that he was surely an angel from heaven.

"Where to?" he asked in a kind voice.

I answered emphatically, "I want to go to heaven!"

The man said, "Wait right here, please," and went inside the store.

A moment later, a couple of police officers spilled out of the store. God's Voice told me not to answer them, and I did not, as they peppered me with questions. They began to grab my arms to handcuff me and I resisted by merely holding my arms together. They soon had me on the ground and handcuffed anyway, and in a few minutes I found myself being loaded into an ambulance.

In my imagination, these people were demons taking me to the pits of hell. Throughout the ambulance ride, God told me to keep my eyes closed if I wanted to be spared, and I heeded these words as if my soul depended upon it. I knew that I was being wheeled into an emergency room by the sounds of doctors and nurses asking me questions, like "Who are you?" and, "Have you taken any drugs?"

Of course, in my mind this was a hospital of nightmarish tortures, which I would endure for eternity if I opened my eyes. The doctors and nurses begged me to talk to them repeatedly; however, I refused.

Then God told me to reveal the answer to the test I had been given which I had written on the notebook; and I did, shouting, "One God!"

I opened my eyes for a moment and saw that the emergency room looked like what I imagined a standard emergency room would look like. They said that if I did not talk to them then they would be forced to stick a needle down my penis to determine what, if any, drugs I might have in my system. After a moment, they realized I was not going to speak to them, and a fire erupted in the vein of my genitals as I felt the needle draining urine away from my bladder. This pain would recur, intermittently, for the next five years. During this time, I never knew when the pain in my penis would strike. This would be but one of the many reminders of all I had experienced in the course of this life-altering week.

The hospital phoned my grandmother after finding her phone number in my wallet. She, in turn, phoned my adopted sister, Kim. Kim happened to be managing a hotel in Tuscaloosa at the time, and she rushed to the emergency room.

Kim was appalled at my disheveled appearance. I could hear the deep concern in her voice as she tried to convince me to speak to her. I remained silent, though, as I could not rule out the possibility that she was another demon, merely masking her voice through magic. I was wheeled away, eyes closed and lips tight, in a rolling bed, down the corridors of the unknown. The last thing I remember was my sister's voice comforting me as I fell unconscious.

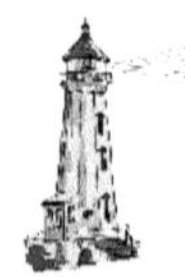

COMING TO

After awaking from a sleep that lasted a thousand years, I found myself lying in a hospital bed. When a black man dressed as an orderly came in and started chatting with me, I remembered God's Voice in the emergency room commanding me not to speak to anyone. In response to this supreme directive I glared at the blue uniformed man in silence.

"You need a bath," he said.

He ushered me into a room dominated by a metallic tub. God's Voice had given me no admonition with regard to following people's instructions, as long as I did not speak. I silently disrobed and entered the steaming water, allowing the man to scrub my shoulders with a sponge and wash my hair.

After the bath, he led me into a small cafeteria where a tray filled with eggs, bacon, and grits was placed before me. At first I refused to eat, remembering God's instructions for me to eat nothing, but to only drink water.

The man gently pried my lips open with a fork full of eggs, and the experience of tasting food for the first time in days was extraordinary. It then struck me that God had sent an angel to me in the guise of this man, in order for me to be allowed to eat.

Immediately, I was chewing the food hungrily, and in a minute even holding the fork myself, shoveling the salty breakfast into my mouth with gusto as my angel beamed. Later that day, my older adopted brothers and sister, David, Bill, and Kim, filed into my room. They were met by a deathly silence, which they couldn't break, no matter how they tried to persuade me.

They were a part of the hodgepodge of families who had adopted me into their lives, following my mother's death. When I was a child they were adolescents, and when I was an adolescent they were in their twenties. These people had been mainstays of my life since I was seven. Prior to this I had followed all of their commands without question. Despite a lifetime of good times and important lessons, my face was now a mask of silence in the face of my family's concerned inquiries.

The look of horror on their faces was clear. They realized I was not going to respond to any of their questions no matter how they cajoled me. Inside, I could feel their frustration, but I was not prepared to break God's direct command for any reason until I had some sense that he was ready for me to do so. I was given medication throughout the day. I swallowed the pills with water unquestioningly, as I was in no position to be anything other than compliant with the wishes of the masters of this new restricted environment.

The behavioral medicine section of Druid City Hospital was divided into three areas of care, organized by the seriousness of the patients' conditions. I was in the section housing the most severe cases, with the most cognitively impaired people. I remember sitting in a rocking chair surrounded by elderly people who were clearly disabled, many of whom would not speak at all, or who were mumbling to themselves. After a time of being surrounded by these gentle souls, I felt as if God at last wanted me to speak.

I pronounced in a loud voice, "God made the voices stop!" I was referring to the chorus of spirits that had compelled me to begin my journey in the first place.

I noticed a psychiatrist sauntering by, who only said, "God works through the medicine."

He continued on his way without breaking stride. Although at this point I knew practically nothing about mental health, what the doctor told me at that moment struck a chord.

I had a scientific mind, and had no problem visualizing my mind as a physical entity, which could be altered through chemical means. What he'd said wasn't a difficult concept for me to grasp. I'd been given some form of medication, and if the medicine did, indeed, help me, then perhaps God did work in more mundane ways than he had recently chosen to demonstrate to me through the Voices. This was an effective nudge back into the more realistic philosophical underpinnings I had maintained before I had a psychotic break with reality.

I started seeing the world more clearly again at this point and enjoyed the rediscovered power of speech. The only other people who were available for me to talk to, at that time, were the severely mentally restricted patients sitting all around, so I began trying to talk to them. They were silent for the most part, or they talked about things that did not make sense to me.

My adopted brothers and sister's eyes beamed with unconcealed relief when I spoke to them at their next visit. I was able to speak to my grandmother on the telephone, since she was too physically disabled to visit me at the hospital. To my surprise, she did not sound completely distraught over my new set of circumstances, but instead spoke more calmly than the other members of my family. After a few days of improvement, I was transferred to the second tier of hospital care where the patients were much more focused on their surroundings.

I felt like I was in the frame of mind I was in before the strange experiences began occurring. I realized that what I had been experiencing was considered a form of mental illness—by the medical professionals. In my mind though, what I had experienced was very real. I had managed to survive the ordeal God had set before me, so I was allowed by this Higher Power to continue with my everyday pattern of life.

I cannot overemphasize the fact that all of this was new to me. I had never been a resident at a hospital, nor had I been surrounded by mental patients. I talked to a man who told me he was a psychologist. He asked me questions that I tried to answer honestly. He later brought my family into a room with me and told us that I had schizophrenia. I found this diagnosis difficult to believe.

I asked the doctor, "Have you ever read the book, 'Future Shock'?"

After thinking a moment he said, "Yes I have."

Future shock was a sociological book I had read in high school which premised that people could become overwhelmed by the sheer volume of technological and societal changes that occur.

I told him, "Maybe what I experienced was all a form of future shock."

He then announced that the meeting was over, without commenting upon my observation.

During the course of the next two weeks, I was bombarded with information about schizophrenia, as well as with the antipsychotic medication, which I was told I would have to take for the rest of my life. I also learned more about the people whose ranks I had joined. Everyone around me was older than me, and for the most part seemed very pleasant. None of them seemed particularly dangerous, though they all seemed to have a glare in their eyes which indicated that they were resigned with their situation.

I could certainly sympathize with their predicament. And while they seemed much like many of the people I knew who were not mentally ill, I didn't believe that I was, in fact, a part of their society. That is, I did not believe that I truly had a mental illness. I thought that maybe I had experienced something temporary like a "nervous breakdown". Over the years I would hear many people with mental illness describe the same mistaken belief. One thing that I knew we all did have in common was the sense of shame for having to be there, separated from the rest of humanity.

As someone new to living with a mental illness, I was accompanied by a stigma that felt almost palpable. Before, the vast majority of people in society did not look at me as "other," and then all of a sudden they did. Nothing stressed this point as much as the steel door that kept me locked in my new restricted environment. It symbolized the fact that I was now separate from the rest of society, if only temporarily. How was I supposed to learn to feel comfortable in my own skin from this point forward, let alone face what other people may think of me? The world outside did not feel comfortable with my presence, and I certainly did not feel comfortable within the confines of this new world. I did not yet feel a kinship with the people with whom I was confined, and did not believe in my heart that they held any answers for me as to how I should carry on with my life.

I felt ashamed because I was not considered strong enough mentally to know what was real and what was not. I felt as if I could not be sure whether other people would be afraid of me because of the new way I was defined. I was very anxious to regain my freedom to move about, although I had no idea what I would do next, except to return home to my grandmother's house.

After two weeks, I was cleared to leave the hospital and I received a bottle of antipsychotic medication called Risperdal to take for the road. Kim's husband, Scott, came by to pick me up from the hospital and take me back to Huntsville. They wished us the best of luck, pointing us in the direction of the mental health center once we made it home. While I was completely free from the psychotic symptoms which had plagued me before my hospitalization, I departed the confines of the Druid City Hospital with a dose of humbling defeat.

After I came home, Bill, one of my aforementioned older adopted siblings, took matters in hand with regard to my mental health care. He worked frantically to get me signed up for mental health services at the Huntsville/Madison County Mental Health Center (HMCMHC), as well as for Social Security benefits. I had a very difficult time acquiring the medication that I needed because it was extremely expensive, and I had no money. I remember looking at the stone face of a grey haired female pharmacy technician who announced that I would not receive my medicine unless I could first produce several hundred dollars. After jumping through many hoops, Bill finally helped to obtain the medication I needed through the HMCMHC, and I resumed taking it immediately.

I thought that Social Security benefits were only for elderly people and had no idea they were available to people with disabilities, including mental illness. Matters were complicated in this area by the fact my grandmother was afraid to accept any money, thinking with certainty that I would have to pay it back. The Social Security Administration telephoned her, and she was at a loss as to how to answer their barrage of questions, such as how much rent I paid, and what kind of property I owned.

"He doesn't pay me any rent," she informed them resolutely.

Soon after this, they began sending my grandmother checks for about two hundred dollars every month, which we were afraid to spend. Grandmother kept the lion's share of these funds in a separate savings account, for fear she would have to return the money later.

I soon discovered that having a mental illness created serious problems for me in the romantic arena. I telephoned the woman I will call Julie, whom I had dated on and off for the past three years, and told her that I had been hospitalized for having a mental illness. She never returned any more of my calls. After a couple weeks of this silent treatment I knew I was in real trouble. Aside from the fact that I had lost any chance of a romantic relationship with the lady I loved, the thought that I might never be able to form a lasting relationship was particularly terrifying. I had only had two sexual partners for short periods of time while attending one of the biggest party schools in the nation. Furthermore, I had been unsuccessful at forming any kind of lasting romantic relationship throughout the course of my life. I had been sustained throughout my young life by thinking it was inevitable that I would eventually form a serious, long-term bond with someone. Now the prospect of love in the future seemed much further out of my reach. I had no idea what further impact having a mental illness might have on my life.

I thought that it would be very difficult for me to return to school and believed that law school was now completely out of the question. I was unsure of myself, and my compass of personal direction was spinning out of control. I thought to myself, "I really don't know how to do anything," since I had never really had to fend for myself. My vision of the future was clouded as I imagined that I might even become homeless when all was said and done.

I knew, for instance, that after studying for years in college, I certainly didn't want to work on an assembly line or wash dishes for minimum wage the rest my life. These were two of the jobs I had done over school vacations, and the prospect of eking out an existence in an environment of backbreaking toil was one vision of the future I simply did not want to face. Bill told me that I was now eligible for Social Security Disability benefits, but to me that sounded too good to be true.

My world was shattered and I did not even know where to begin to pick up the pieces. I soon decided that taking medication was not a solution and stopped taking it. I did not believe that I had a mental illness, and the medication tethered me symbolically to this new world of despair and uncertainty.

Bill, David, and Kim insisted quite forcefully that I should resume taking the medication. Immediately. They said if I simply took a pill, that I would never again have to experience the nightmare scenario I described earlier. But I soon found out that matters were certainly not so simple. For one thing, the medicine had a number of side effects, which I found particularly disconcerting. One of these side effects was dry mouth, a condition where my mouth was completely dry of saliva. I never really appreciated how important saliva is to digestion and overall level of comfort until it had vanished from my mouth entirely.

When I tried to enjoy a meal with Bill and his family after resuming my medication regimen, I was unable to taste any of the food. I didn't understand that this side effect would go away in time, and the prospect of never being able to enjoy food again, was immensely frightening. Why it didn't occur to the doctor to inform me that this side effect was temporary remains a mystery.

Blurred vision was another temporary side effect that occurred soon after resuming the medicine. I did not remember having this side effect or the dry mouth when I first began taking the medication at the hospital. I had no way of knowing it would be temporary. These side effects, combined with my initial reluctance to face the fact that I would need my medicine, prompted me to quit taking my medication again after a couple of weeks.

There was one part of me that thought everything that I had experienced had been real, and another part of me that thought that I had just had a nervous breakdown and did not really have a mental illness. To my way of thinking, a nervous breakdown was much more impermanent than the chronic condition of living with a serious mental illness.

I was not experiencing the same psychotic symptoms, but there was a total lack of energy which was a completely new experience in my life. Sometimes I would stay in bed all day and all night in an effort to make myself sleep. I did not want to have to be conscious and think about the seemingly unsolvable nature of my new problems. Unable to slumber throughout the day or much at night, I felt hopeless and found myself sleeping for only three hours. It was not long before these intense feelings of hopelessness left me pondering the notion of suicide. "How good it would be," I thought, "to sleep forever and never have to worry about what I should do with my life."

I realize today that what I was experiencing was the post-psychotic depression that often occurs after a person has a break with reality.

After a few days, I decided that it would be for the best if I could simply end my life. I owned many firearms. My stepfather was an avid gun owner and had given them to me over the years. I called my friend

Tommy and told him, "I'm thinking about just taking one of my rifles and using it to blow my brains out."

"Don't do it, Jim," he said. "You'll really break my heart if you do."

Later on, as my hand caressed the wooden stock of the rifle in my bedroom that I thought could instantly transport me away from my problems, I thought about what Tommy had said and visualized what one of the bullets would do to my head. I thought of what my grandmother would see when she walked into the bedroom and found my body, and it was something I was just not willing to make her go through. On the other hand, I thought, all of my problems would be over if I could simply go to sleep and never wake up.

I grabbed an entire bottle of sleeping pills, known as Ativan, thinking that I would never wake up after I took them. "The world will be better off without me," I thought, as I prepared to drift off into an eternal slumber. "No one will have to worry about how to help me take care of myself" I thought, as I swallowed the entire bottle of the sleep remedy. I slept for a time and awakened to the somewhat surprising realization that I was still alive. I didn't know how or why I was still breathing, but assumed that for some reason the amount of medication I downed was not enough to finish the job. It was not a complete surprise that I awoke to consciousness, because there was always a part of me that knew this was not a sure means of death.

With consciousness, all the fear and uncertainty about my future returned. I caught a ride to Huntsville Hospital and told the hospital staff what I had done, in a desperate kind of plea for them to come up with some kind of remedy for the feeling of desperation I felt. I stayed in the psychiatric ward of Huntsville Hospital for a few days, but I discovered that the hospital was not a cure-all. And besides, the hospital staff did not seem particularly enthusiastic about having me there at all. Through sighs and shrugs at key moments, they left me with the impression that I did not have enough wrong with me to be in the hospital. When I was released, I was more uncertain than ever about what to do to escape the ever-darkening cloud of despair surrounding me.

I settled into a routine of watching television with my grandmother and rarely leaving the house. I wasn't eating much because no food interested me, and I was shedding pounds rapidly. I was reluctant to talk to any of my old friends because I was so ashamed about what had happened and what I felt I had become. Before, I had been a young man bent on success, with enough drive to become a straight "A" student and ride a bicycle across the country. Now, I felt that I had become completely directionless, and was not even sure how I would earn enough money to pay for food and shelter. I did not have the kind of parents who could provide for me for the better part of my life, in case of some calamity. I had a grandmother in her 80's and an elderly stepfather who, in everyone's opinion, had done more than enough for my family and for me already. I had spent the past four years feeling like I was on a set timetable for becoming not only independent, but in a position to be of real financial assistance to my grandmother. This new wrinkle to my life's circumstances left me feeling as if I was in more jeopardy than ever, in terms of creating a responsible life for myself, in a limited amount of time.

I began seeing a therapist at the HMCMHC, named Marilyn. She was in her late thirties and very attractive, in a businesslike fashion. She had short brown hair and a smile that conveyed friendly warmth and concern. She explained that what I had experienced was a symptom of my mental illness called psychosis.

"Psychosis means that you experience sensations of hearing or seeing things that are not there. These are called hallucinations. Some people even smell and feel things that are not there. It can also mean having beliefs that do not correspond with the evidence at hand. These illogical beliefs are called delusions."

She explained that the public sometimes confuse the word "psychotic" with the word "psychopathic," and that people who have been psychotic were no more dangerous than people who did not experience such symptoms. "Psychopathic" was the term used to define people who did not appear to have a conscience, such as serial murderers. The two states of mind were not connected. She explained other facts about schizophrenia and made sure I understood how important it was for me to take my medication, to ensure that my psychotic symptoms did not return.

Despite her impassioned pleas that I take my medication, I continued secretly to dispose of the pills. I felt guilty about concealing the truth from Marilyn that I was reluctant to take my medication, since

I valued our therapeutic relationship. I felt that I could be open with Marilyn about practically every aspect of my life and was grateful that I had someone with whom I could discuss the fact that I had no idea what direction my life would take. Marilyn was the only person who could convey a genuine knowledge of what I was going through, combined with a genuine sense of concern for my wellbeing. When you add to this mix a kind of hard-won wisdom of the world and an ability to never lose control of her emotions, then what you end up with is the perfect recipe for the type of person I needed in my life at that time. In many ways, Marilyn reminded me of a much younger version of my grandmother. She had been in business in the marketing department at the Huntsville Airport before deciding to leave that behind to attain her Master's Degree in Counseling Psychology, and eventually becoming a Licensed Professional Counselor. She also had a tendency to speak in the same soothing, mellow tones in which my grandmother communicated.

She recommended a program called Day Treatment as a way to learn more about living with a mental illness. Day treatment was a four-hour program for three to five days per week, where people with serious mental illnesses gathered to learn coping skills and training for managing their symptoms. The people with whom I attended Day Treatment were far older than I, and seemed to function at a much lower level than I did. Many of them appeared endlessly distracted by their symptoms, and they talked to themselves constantly. Others seemed to have much lower I.Q.'s than average. Some of the attendees had a disheveled appearance.

Attending Day Treatment and seeing how much more psychiatrically disabled the people there were served to strengthen my belief that there was a fundamental difference between other people diagnosed with a mental illness and myself. I felt that the doctors and various professionals must have made a mistake in suggesting that I was in the same situation as the others in this group.

Marilyn explained to me that I was just like the average person when I was not in a psychotic state, but that if I didn't take my medicine I would continue to have psychotic breaks with reality, and that each additional break would leave me worse off than before. She explained that the medication I took was only a few years old, and that the people

I was in group with had not had the advantage of the scientific breakthroughs made in that area. They had been diagnosed with schizophrenia many years before the medication that was available to me had been discovered by medical researchers.

"This is why the 1990's are known as the decade of the brain," she said with a knowing smile.

The medications people took before often caused as many problems as they solved. The older medications could eliminate positive symptoms associated with schizophrenia, such as hallucinations and delusions. However they usually made the negative symptoms much worse, which included feelings of depression and a lack of motivation.

Most patients had begun taking the newer medications once they were widely available, but by that point all of the damage had been done. Some continued to remain on the older medications, since their bodies could not adjust to the breakthrough medications. Although I listened seriously to what she had to say and intellectually understood it, I did not come to a point where I really believed, wholeheartedly, that I was similar to my group members. The seriousness of the situation I was in was made clear to me by the people surrounding me in therapy group, though, and I realized that if my calculations were wrong that I could end up just as seriously disabled as they.

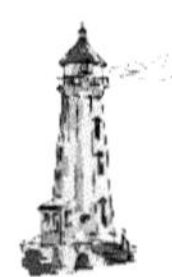

MOVING FORWARD

I attended Day Treatment for about one week before deciding that I never wanted to return. My grandmother was content to let me stay at home with her without demanding that I return to the program. The look of dejection that she saw on my face after Day Treatment convinced her as much as anything I said to her.

It was now nearing the end of the summer in which I had been diagnosed with schizophrenia. I took another overdose of Ativan, which I chased with alcohol this time to increase the likelihood of my own death. Following my overdose, I began wandering the streets of my neighborhood because I did not want my grandmother to find my dead body. I walked a couple of miles to a hospital where I fainted and they took me in, thinking I had suffered heat exhaustion.

When I made the blunder of telling my grandmother that I had actually tried to take my own life, I could see the intense look of hurt in her eyes. She must have remembered how my mother died in her sleep and felt the flood of remembered emotion from that traumatic event. This was certainly not my intention, and it increased my feelings of guilt about the entire situation. I thought to myself, "Why was I even born?"

Grandmother asked my stepfather to remove all of my firearms from the house, which he did. I continued my malaise, watching television, not sleeping much, not eating much, and leaving home infrequently.

There was conflict between me and my extended family members over the issue of my medications. They, along with my therapist, were very insistent that I take the medication as prescribed, while I was reluctant to take it. Grandmother asked that I take the medication but was not insistent on the matter.

On one occasion, Bill caught me flushing my medication down the commode. I was brought before an elderly nurse at the HMCMHC who said she had a solution. None of the nurses at the HMCMHC wore uniforms, and their stern looks were the only thing that differentiated them from the other staff. She said that I was to receive an injection of the older medication called Prolixin.

She told me she was going to give me a shot in the buttocks.

"After this, you won't have to worry about medication again for another month," she explained as I was trying to figure out why people were now speaking to me as if I were a child.

Reluctantly, I agreed to the painful prick of the thick needle required to deliver the syrupy elixir to my system.

"That wasn't so bad, was it?" she said.

"I guess not," I replied, with an expression that was now as severe as hers.

It was a week later when the living nightmare began.

Sometime in the morning while sitting at my grandmother's house, I began to feel my body tremble all over. What made this sensation particularly unsettling was that I was trembling not only on the outside of my body, but on the inside as well. The feelings would not stop no matter what I did, and it was the most uncomfortable sensation, lasting for an extended period of time, that I have ever experienced. David drove me to the emergency room, where I was told by a young male doctor that I should stop taking the Prolixin because I was having an adverse reaction to it. I was given an oral medication to help me get over the reaction more quickly, and was told that my tremors would go away whenever the Prolixin left my bloodstream. The Prolixin didn't leave my system right away, and the constant trembling on my insides only seemed to get worse. After another week of this anguish, thoughts of suicide flooded my mind more forcefully than ever.

I was distressed at the loss of my firearms, which were my one sure method of suicide. I searched my mind for some other certain means to end my suffering.

Concerns about what anyone's reaction would be to finding my remains completely vanished as the pulsating discomfort continued to throb throughout my body. Even if the discomforting vibrations disappeared entirely, I did not wish to remain in a universe where I had to deal with one strange and unforeseen calamity after the next.

If I'd had access to a firearm at that time, there is little doubt that I would no longer be among the living. I was angry with myself for not using one of the weapons to end my life when I'd had the chance.

The next best way to end my life swiftly and surely was with my automobile. I thought that if I could only drive my car into something at a very high speed, then the crash would surely kill me. I would even have the bonus of not having to worry about what people would think of me having committed suicide, since it would look like an accident.

The only thing I could think to drive into was a telephone pole. The problem with that was that all the telephone poles were up on curbs and not easily accessible. I was afraid that I would not hit the pole cleanly. My worst nightmare was that I would survive the wreck only to become even more disabled and in a higher degree of pain.

This fear was enough to unscrew the courage I had fixed in my mind to ram my car into something. As my days passed in contemplation of my own end, the side effects of the medication slowly began to fade. As the physical anguish disappeared, so did the urge to end my life in such a violent fashion.

The summer passed and turned into fall as I isolated myself at my grandmother's house, ruminating about my future. Gradually, I began considering the prospect of completing my college degree. I needed to pass about four more classes in order to graduate, and Kim offered to allow me to live with her, rent free, in Tuscaloosa for the spring semester. In her mind, it was fate that allowed her to live in Tuscaloosa at the exact time I became ill, and she was in a perfect position to help facilitate my graduation. Her only conditions were that I take my medicine as prescribed and see a therapist at the Indian Rivers Community Mental Health Center in Tuscaloosa until I could return to the care of Marilyn upon graduation. With that goal in mind, it was far easier to make it through the fall without thoughts of suicide.

I visited my sister in Tuscaloosa once before the spring semester began, and one of my friends, named Ryan, commented upon how much weight I had lost.

"Wow, Jim, you look really great!"

"Thanks Ryan," I said, with my eyes downcast. "I haven't been eating all that much lately."

"Well you look really great, Jim!" he smiled.

His girlfriend and several other women from school joined us, and the good company really sparked my appetite. I ate a dish of chicken potpie rapaciously, really enjoying my food for the first time in months. From then on, I ate with the fervor I had before my psychotic break. It was not long before my new slim physique was replaced with the heavyset one I had maintained throughout most of my college career.

I moved in with Kim and her husband, Scott, and began work on finishing my degree in American Studies. This was a far different experience than my previous academic life. Before, I was constantly surrounded by parties and mingled with people my own age on a regular basis. Now, I was content to stay at home, even on weekends. I did a number of chores, including helping with the yard work, keeping my room clean, and helping with dinner, all of which I had never been expected to do at grandmother's house.

I was extremely uncertain about my ability to maintain good grades and successfully graduate. It had only been about six months since I had been diagnosed with schizophrenia. My life before my diagnosis, which had been free of doubts about my own capabilities, now seemed like a separate lifetime. I didn't think that the Jim who had ridden the bicycle across the country had a life anything like this new Jim, struggling with serious mental illness.

While recovering in Huntsville from my psychotic break with reality, I initially had a much more difficult time reading than I'd had prior to my illness. My therapist taught me that this was not uncommon and that I could work to build my reading ability back up to its previous level, even if I had to start with one line of text per day.

Probably the most helpful technique I discovered for remedying this situation was to listen to books on tape. My therapist gave me a book to read called *The Quiet Room: A Journey out of the Torment of Madness*, written by Lori Schiller and Amanda Bennett, about Lori Schiller, who was in recovery from schizophrenia.

When I had a difficult time concentrating on it, I told her that I could not read it. Later, I found the book on tape at the public library and discovered that it was much simpler for me to listen to a reading of the book, instead. I listened to other books on tape, which I found enjoyable, and it became a transition into reading books with my own eyes again.

Though I had built up my ability to read written material to a point that I could read a simple novel, I was still quite unsure of my ability to process and analyze the complex information that would be required to pass college courses. I was also fearful that even if I passed my classes, I would fundamentally change my grade point average by making all C's or D's.

I also didn't have the same zeal for the social interaction required in learning as I did before becoming ill. Following my return to college, I rarely if ever spoke up in class, which was something for which I had previously been renowned. Before my illness, I often surprised myself with the kinds of inspired insights I could reach in the course of a lecture. One of the American studies graduate students who had befriended me nicknamed me Jim Jones, after the infamous cult leader from the seventies, because I spoke with such relish. I just didn't think speaking up in class was as important as I did before my illness, and I was more insecure about my ability to reason.

When a person is diagnosed with a mental illness, often the emotions that occur surrounding the illness are more damaging than the actual symptoms. A person diagnosed with schizophrenia is likely to have intense feelings of insecurity. Often, these feelings can lead people to extreme isolation because they don't know if the world at large will accept them for who they are. They feel as if they are walking around with this fundamental flaw on the inside that, if revealed, will drive other people away from them. They fear that people will reject them even if they don't know they have a mental illness because of any apparent differences the illness may bring about. These fears feed upon themselves and are fueled even further by the palpable fright and disregard that many people in the greater society have for People Living with Mental Illnesses (PLMI).

Despite my fears of not being able to handle college classes, and thanks to the positive family environment offered by Kim and her husband, Scott, I managed to maintain the high grades that I had before I was diagnosed with my mental illness. In the spring of 1997, I graduated from the UA. Although seeing me graduate from college was one of my grandmother's greatest goals in life, she was 82 years old and too disabled to witness the actual ceremony.

After graduation, I moved back home with my grandmother in Huntsville. At this point, I lacked the confidence to apply for law school and decided to look for a job. I had absolutely no experience in finding a career and had not taken advantage of the College Career Center in Tuscaloosa while I had still lived there. I felt directionless in my quest to find work, and ended up applying for jobs in many fields. After a couple of months of this fumbling approach to finding work, I finally landed a job as a front desk clerk at a Holiday Inn in Huntsville.

I was not taking any medication for my mental illness and had stopped attending my appointments at the HMCMHC all-together. I thought that what I had experienced when I was diagnosed was some kind of temporary phenomenon and that I was no longer affected by mental illness. During this time, I spent a lot of time driving back and forth to Tuscaloosa to socialize with my friend, Tommy, who had not yet graduated. My level of self-confidence increased dramatically as I spent time with Tommy and his circle of friends. My psychotic break from reality became more of a distant memory since I didn't experience any return of the symptoms I had before. While I continued to have problems forming romantic relationships, my prospects in this area seemed much improved and my outlook was much more optimistic.

One blemish on this outlook of optimism was the sizeable amount of debt I had accrued in college. The greatest amount I owed, by far, was for hospital bills. There were many times when I was admitted to the hospital, and was not covered by insurance, or the insurance I had did not cover medical bills associated with my mental illness. My new job was only part-time and it didn't pay nearly enough to cover the amount of money I owed. In the area of finances, as in so many other matters, I was inexperienced. Problems with medical bills and other debts continued to plague me.

While living with my grandmother during this time, I watched a lot of television. It was an episode of the Oprah show that inspired me to start doing some walking during my free time. I decided to try it and see what happened. I began walking around my grandmother's neighborhood for thirty minutes, and eventually for hour-long intervals. I discovered that it was greatly invigorating. After a month or so, I could really see a difference in my waistline and enjoyed the favorable comments I received from my co-workers. The realization that physical fitness was a palace with an open gate and not one with high walls spurred me to continue exercising. My level of self-esteem was heightened even more by this accomplishment.

During walks, I would experience a state of euphoria at times, and I found that I had increased creativity. Lyrics to songs would form miraculously in my mind during these hikes, and I had particular clarity of thought and enough time to consider how to plan my future. It was during one of these exercises that my original dream of attending law school was rekindled.

If I began attending the UASL in the fall of the next year, I would have only deviated from my original plan by one year! My earlier lack of faith in my abilities was banished and I began pondering how to make my dream a reality. It had been about a year and a half since I had been hospitalized. This gave me about six months to take the steps necessary to be accepted to law school for the fall.

I enrolled in a study course for taking the test required for potential law students, called the Law School Administration Test (LSAT). I was provided study materials, which I spent hours going over. The UASL was extremely competitive and I would need to score as highly as I could on the LSAT in order to be admitted.

The entire application process created a great deal of additional stress in my life. I worked frantically to collect everything I would need, including recommendation letters from professors.

In the midst of this process, an unexpected visitor from the past made an abrupt entrance back into my life. My older brother, Bert, showed up at the townhouse where my grandmother and I lived. He was bedraggled and had nowhere to live. He made his purpose clear to me that he had every intention of living with my grandmother and me at the house.

This would be the first time that Bert had lived with me since I was seven years old, though it would not be the first time he had lived with my grandmother. During the spring break of my senior year in college, five months before my first psychotic break with reality, I returned home to discover that Bert had been living with Grandmother for months while I was away at school. He was not living there upon my return for spring break because, as my grandmother told me, he was now a resident in the city jail after attempting to shoplift saw blades from the local Wal-Mart.

All of this began when Bert lost his job at a concrete manufacturing plant, where he had labored for years. He had failed a mandatory drug screen. Bert then resided with grandmother while taking substance abuse recovery classes in order to treat his addiction to marijuana. While in the classes, Bert continued to abuse drugs and eventually spiraled down so far that he ended up behind bars.

Grandmother told me that it was now my duty to visit Bert in jail. I had never been to a jail and didn't know what to expect. I brought Bert coffee, soap, and a few other items he would need while incarcerated. The older brother I saw in jail seemed far different from the man I remembered from the time I had seen him at the last family Christmas, his six-foot-four inch frame far thinner and more disheveled. Seven years my senior, Bert had earned a bachelor's degree in marketing from the University of Alabama in Huntsville. I had asked him on previous occasions why he did not try to utilize his degree to attain employment other than sweating it out at the factory, but never received a definitive answer.

After this family reunion, I returned to school to begin the fall semester with a heavy mind. Grandmother assured me, though, that Bert would not be allowed to move back in with her. Within six months I experienced my first psychotic break with reality, which I have already described to you.

A year and a half following that break with reality, Bert's return felt very much like a hostile takeover. I pleaded with my grandmother to insist he stay somewhere else. I also did my best to explain to Bert why his residing in the house simply would not work. Bert ignored all my protests and so did my grandmother. Despite my pleas to the contrary, Bert became a permanent resident in our home.

From the outset of this new and unexpected arrangement, something became immediately apparent to me: I did not have to speak to Bert for more than a few sentences to tell that he clearly had a mental illness. He would describe in a ceaseless flow of words how frightening it was that there were satellites in space that could read people's minds. He knew that unknown people for uncertain reasons had bugged the apartment he had previously occupied. He was grandiosely religious, thinking that God sent him messages through both subtle and direct means, whether it was through songs on the radio or in the way sunlight splashed on the kitchen counter. In trying to disprove to Bert that what he was thinking was unreasonable, I found it difficult because what he was describing couldn't be disproved. Certainly, he had no evidence to support what he was proclaiming, aside from the circumstantial bits his mind had managed to string together.

Years later, I read a passage from G. K. Chesterton's pro-Christianity essay, "Orthodoxy," which quite accurately describes this phenomenon. Chesterton attempts to show how trying to argue against Christianity is akin to a form of what he calls "madness." In doing so, he described the types of arguments that people who are "mad" make. Although Bert was extremely intelligent, he was unable to break out of what Chesterton calls circular logic. Indeed, most of the many people I have known with mental illness are extremely spiritual in nature. Many times, they are simply unable to perceive what it is they experience because they have a chemical imbalance. This conflicts with the image portrayed by the media in the public's eye. Those with mental illness are portrayed as dangerous "psycho killers," incapable of having spiritual concerns. Movies and television shows tend to depict PLMI in a negative light in order to increase viewership. News broadcasts also engage in this activity by only discussing PLMI when something horrible has happened. The millions upon millions of other PLMI who are gentle in temperament go unnoticed. This ratings game is extremely detrimental to the image of PLMI as a whole.

Bert's symptoms aside, it was evident that he was capable and willing to provide personal care for my grandmother. Right away, he began preparing all of her meals. He also performed, without hesitation, any maintenance that he could handle on the house. Aside from being one of the most intelligent people I have ever known, my brother is the hardest working person I have ever known, and he jumped into the duties of Grandmother's care with gusto. His perseverance in this respect carried some weight, I suppose, in my grandmother's decision to allow him to remain. This, combined with her seemingly infinite capacity to care about the welfare of others, especially her children, meant that Bert had her permission to stay.

My stepfather, Dave, paid the mortgage, since he actually owned the house. I urged him to acknowledge that Bert clearly had some form of mental illness, but he stayed uninvolved in the activities in the house. Like me, he really didn't know what to do.

I recall one night in particular when I was upstairs in my room in the townhouse. I could hear my brother downstairs screaming incessantly from some hallucinations or delusions. I telephoned my stepfather and described to him what was going on and explained that I was really frightened. He said that if things got out of hand I should call the police. He was seventy-two years old at this point. He had also had a tremendous amount of experience trying to care for my mother, who had suffered from schizophrenia. That had ended badly, and it was likely that he just did not have the energy or experience to try to deal with a similar situation again.

There was a mistrust of mental health in general that seemed to pervade my family. This mistrust stemmed from the perceived lack of care that my mother received while she was ill, which culminated in the loss of her children and her eventual death.

I believe that my grandmother and stepfather were, in part, convinced that neither my brother nor I had a mental illness, despite the clear evidence to the contrary. Indeed, my stepfather was considered rather eccentric by many people, in that he bought his clothes from the Salvation Army and insisted on driving cars older than almost anyone on his level of income would have driven. In a way, he may have thought Bert was simply expressing his own eccentricity by refusing to take advantage of his education and living his life as a vagabond. I telephoned my adopted brothers, David and Bill, describing the horrific circumstances that were going on in the house, hoping that they had some instantaneous solution to remedy the situation. They, too, were at a loss as to what I should do.

I spent a great deal of time and an enormous amount of energy trying to convince my brother that what he was experiencing was related to symptoms of mental illness. I continued to believe that I did not have schizophrenia in any major way, since I clearly was not experiencing what Bert was. I thought that since I could grasp the concept of it being an illness, I could hold any similar manifestations of the illness at bay simply by willing myself to do so. I also felt I could do it without any need to take medication. I thought to myself, "If I don't really have a mental illness, taking medication will only cause me more problems."

At this point I didn't have any access to medication, anyway, since I had cut ties with my only source of the medication—the HMCMHC.

With the stress of this situation, combined with continued concerns about being accepted to law school, something strange and unexpected happened. Incessantly listening to Bert's explanations of how God makes his wishes clear through haphazard signs and how men could read other men's minds through satellite-powered methods, it began to take a heavy toll. The symptom-induced ravings of Bert slowly began to take on a greater air of reality.

The many irons I now had in the fire began to burn with an intensity fueled by my brother's delusional arguments. This never ending cycle of frenetic activity and debate began affecting my own fragile psyche. As anyone with experience with mental illness might predict, and indeed, as my therapist had foretold, thoughts and concepts slowly began to unravel for me once again. This time it was in concert with the many psychotic symptoms Bert manifested. The year and a half I had spent trying to come to grips with my first psychotic break was merely the calm before the storm. Soon, the nightmarish psychotic symptoms I had experienced before would be snowballing, and my life would once more be out of my control.

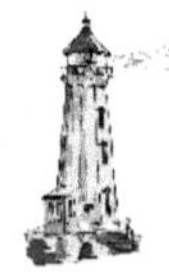

THE ENDLESS APPLICATION

Prior to taking the LSAT, a high school acquaintance that had already been accepted to the UASL stopped by my grandmother's house and gave me some pointers on the application process. He told me to take particular care in how I wrote the letter describing why I should be accepted to law school. He had made a reasonably high score on the LSAT. However, he thought that he had been accepted because of the quality of his letter; he knew another candidate with identical marks who was not accepted.

I was going to bars from time to time, both in Huntsville where I lived with my grandmother and Bert, and when I drove to Tuscaloosa. I ran into some old acquaintances at these watering holes, and I also met some new ones. People could feel the excitement when I described my plans for law school. At one point, I ran into a pretty blonde woman who I had dated a few times prior to my first psychotic break with reality. She told me to give her a call when I started law school. I felt even more eager and determined to attain this goal. Thoughts of all the women who might want to date me increased my drive, as I had always dreamed of being the man all the ladies wanted.

Another person I met on one of these outings in Huntsville told me that he had graduated from the UASL and had started at a job making so much money that he was easily able to pay off his student loans within a year. My whole future would be decided by this test, and I was on edge as I made my way to the examination.

I took the test in a large auditorium filled with people. When I entered the auditorium, I happened to see one of my friends who was re-taking the test because he had not made an acceptable score. We chatted for a few minutes about how awfully difficult the test was, and then we proceeded to sit for the examination. Excitement pervaded the room as the law school hopefuls sat down to compete with one another for the best score. Nerves tingled as I tightly gripped one of the two #2 pencils we were instructed to bring with us. A nervous silence filled the hall as the start of the test was announced.

The test questions seemed more difficult than the practice questions I had studied at home, so I did the best I could to answer them correctly in the allotted time. I left the test feeling a sense of accomplishment that I had completed a step toward reaching my goal and hoped that I had scored high enough to be accepted to the state's most competitive law school.

It was not long before I learned my score. I used a touchtone telephone at Tommy's apartment to access an automated service. I had not scored as well as I had hoped—but I had not scored as low as some of the others applying to the UASL. I had scored well enough to be admitted to many other law schools, even if I was not admitted to my first choice.

My hopes were somewhat bruised with regard to my score on the LSAT, and I called Kim, who had allowed me to live with her during my last semester to tell her about my score. She encouraged me and said that she was proud of me no matter how I scored on the test. With my confidence still shaken, I redoubled my efforts to complete, to perfection, the other parts of the application.

My efforts were disrupted by an event that occurred the day after I took the test. I had a bout of celebratory drinking which led to a nasty hangover. I soon learned that a bad hangover affects driving just about as seriously as being intoxicated.

I was driving a fast, gold-painted Nissan that my stepfather had bought for me. It was the nicest car I had ever owned. However, it was a stick shift, and I was used to driving an automatic. In retrospect, I could see that the stop light I had driven through had indeed changed to red. Before this vision replayed before my eyes, I saw a quarter ton pickup truck bearing down on my car and then slamming into the side of it, spinning it several times.

I was not seriously hurt except from the shock of the impact. My car, however, was totally demolished. The man driving the quarter ton pickup truck and wearing a trucker's cap appeared to be particularly relieved that I had not been more seriously injured. His truck was slightly damaged, and he drove off after the police report was filed. He seemed little interested in the insurance money that I assured him he would collect.

With my freedom of mobility restricted, I then had to figure out how to carry on with my job at the Holiday Inn and how to continue my vital application to the UASL. A surprising figure came to my rescue in this matter; Bert happened to have an extra car on hand.

The car he gave me was a 1979 Monte Carlo that was so light blue in color that it appeared white. It did not run well, however, and it was certainly inappropriate for my excursions back and forth to Tuscaloosa. In spite of that, I thought the car had a cool character, and I even arranged to have an eight-track tape player installed in it. Listening to seventies music in a seventies model car, I floated down the road in mellow style.

I telephoned my stepbrother, Wendell, who was practicing law in St. Louis, and informed him I was applying to law school, had taken the LSAT, but had not scored as well as I would have liked.

His response was, "So you take the test again, until you score what you need."

I said he was right, although there was certainly no more time to take the test before the school year began. Even if there were, I felt I needed more time to prepare. Additionally, I did not have the money to take the test right away.

Around that time, I watched Stephen Spielberg's classic movie, *Dual,* for the first time on television. In *Dual*, a man driving a Dodge Duster is being chased to the death by an unseen person driving an eighteen-wheeler. I felt like the man in the Dodge Duster. I was doing everything I could to escape the inevitable cruelty of life, which was represented by the goliath on eighteen wheels. Poverty, illness, and unforeseen calamity were chasing me down and I was doing everything in my power to escape their relentless pursuit. Painstakingly, I acquired letters of recommendation from past professors, one of which was the man I encountered during my first psychotic break. I had told him there was one God and raved about the fact that I thought his daughter was dating the professor who taught the Twin Peaks class. He was much more cooperative now that I was not in a psychotic state of mind.

While working on my application, I began attending the Twickenham Church of Christ, where I had been baptized when I was twelve years old. The church was unique in that it evolved to be fairly liberal, for its denomination. As far as I know, it is the only liberal-slanting Church of Christ in North Alabama. At any rate, a liberal Church of Christ is still a little stricter than most other churches.

When I reconnected with the church I had stopped attending as a teenager, it added a great deal of meaning to my life. I learned things about Christianity and its virtues in private discussions with the preacher. A liberalized version of the religion of my childhood seemed to be in perfect alignment with my spiritual needs. Once, I invited Bert to attend church with me. This seemed to be in accordance with what I thought God wanted me to do, since Bert talked non-stop about religion, even if most of it was blended with his own delusional ideas. Bert had a somewhat ragged appearance. I really felt tense about him accompanying me among the finely-dressed Sunday morning service congregants. Bert continued to have his own ideas regarding the spiritual realm despite his attendance with me at the Sunday Services. Fortunately, his hallucinations and delusions did not cause him to act inappropriately while in the worship service.

This story took a bizarre turn when I wrote the letter explaining why I should be accepted to the UASL. The first rough draft began as any other such letter would. The stress of the situation, however, continued to grind at my psyche, as well as did the ravings of my now ever-present brother. As I rushed to finish my letter before the due date, I found myself thinking more and more about religion. This renewed spiritual awareness, combined with previous psychotic experiences deeply rooted in religion, slowly but inexorably began to shape the application letter as I wrote it.

It was more than just a letter stating why I wanted to attend law school. It became, instead, a dissertation on my attempt to prove the existence of God and his importance in all of our lives. I seriously doubt that the people making the decision to accept my application were particularly moved to permit my admittance based on this work, despite the fact that it was inspired writing. It was certainly different from what they were looking for in someone aspiring to become a lawyer.

My focus now was more on spiritual matters than on the earthly matters necessary for competent legal practice. I felt compelled to turn in the paper, despite knowing the consequences of turning in a letter that was clearly not what they were looking for. My application was completed, and there was nothing for me to do other than to wait for the outcome and to keep working at my job.

As it turned out, the head of the committee who oversaw admission decisions to UASL that year happened to be someone I was well acquainted with. I had met him on the first day of his professorship at the law school a few years earlier on the day I began my copier's assistant job there.

He was a distinguished black man who had left a successful practice in California to become a law professor in the Deep South. We seemed to get along right away, and I had occasion to talk to him in his office from time to time. Once, he was even a guest lecturer in an American Studies Class. The subject had been the Civil Rights Movement. The book he spoke about was a very interesting one which looked at the Civil Rights Movement in an "outside the box" way. I was pleased to find out that this man was the head of the committee for determining who would be selected for admittance since I was acquainted with him more than with any other professor at the school. It will come as little surprise to most to know that this man was one of the positive Voices in my head during my first psychotic trial, discussed earlier in this work.

I arranged a meeting with him. I would have done this anyway, even if he had not been the head of the determination committee, in order to talk about my application. We were not far into our conversation when the professor told me rather forcefully that I should write a book. Perhaps he was impressed by the strength of my writing, even if he thought I had used it in the wrong context.

When I began asking him about my chances of being accepted to law school, he asked me in turn if it was really my dream to become a lawyer. This question surprised me, but what surprised me even more, was that I had no answer for him. To become a lawyer had certainly been my goal for the last four years. I certainly craved the prestige and money that came along with the profession. I knew that many lawyers actually had very high ideals, in terms of the social service they could provide others. My stepbrother, Wendell, for example worked to help consumers file bankruptcies and made very little profit from his profession in helping others. This idea was appealing more and more as my sense of spirituality heightened; however, I could not tell this man that being a lawyer was actually my dream! This state of affairs came as more of a surprise to me than it probably did to him.

"It's something I would like to accomplish, in any event," I told him.

He responded by saying, "I wanted to become a lawyer throughout my childhood and worked diligently to reach my dreams."

I knew that he had grown up in a home with very few monetary resources and had overcome a number of serious obstacles in order to reach his goals.

We went on to talk about the various distractions that plague young law students, and he informed me that I should probably apply to a number of law schools instead of the highly competitive UASL, if law school was really something I wanted to pursue. I couldn't make a compelling argument to my friend for why I should be admitted to the program.

Perhaps this was as good a reason as any for me not to be admitted. A lawyer's job is to persuade a jury, and I was incapable of persuading my own ally as to why I should be admitted to his law school. My own off topic application was testament to my lack of focus on the letter of the law.

I left the meeting feeling somewhat disconcerted yet somehow comforted by the fact that the professor clearly thought I had the ability to write a book. I knew I was a good writer, yet somehow the notion of writing a book seemed far removed from what I was capable of, at that time. It took many years to develop to a point where this dream came to fruition.

After that fateful conversation with the professor, however, I lived my life with the knowledge that I was capable of writing at least one book that would benefit the people who read it.

Since that time, I have discovered a genuine and altogether different dream from that of becoming a lawyer or a writer—and I have fulfilled it! It took many years more in my journey for this to happen, and most people would be surprised that it became my true dream, rather than that of becoming a lawyer. The making of this dream, and how it came into existence as a reality, will be described much further in this work.

I continued to drive back and forth to Tuscaloosa. However, these repeated commutes eventually took their toll on the car my brother had given me, and it finally died completely on one of my trips into Tuscaloosa.

When it happened, I was not instantly connected with the rest of the world by a cellular phone. In 1998, I am sure that there were many people who had cell phones; however, the technology was completely alien, to me. I knew just enough about cell phones to know they were probably something I could not afford.

I was within a mile of the brand-new Mercedes plant outside Tuscaloosa when the car's engine blew out. My friend Tommy's brother-in-law happened to be an engineer at the plant, so I did things the pre-cell-phone way and walked to the plant where Tommy's brother-in-law was kind enough to allow me to use his cell phone—who I called, I do not remember. Tommy had graduated and was no longer living in Tuscaloosa, and I had been staying with a friend who did not have a car. This meant that I now had no car and had no way of getting a ride home to Huntsville.

My level of mental stress heightened as I spent the next few days trying to figure out what I should do to make it back home. I began walking all over Tuscaloosa in an effort to make sense of what I should do without wheels.

At one point I spoke to a man with a salt and pepper beard wearing a doo rag at a used car dealership. He took me on a test drive of a shiny red American car, in which he spoke to me of his troubles dating a dancer at a strip club.

"You don't go to strip clubs do you?" he asked me with a scrutinizing glare.

"Why, heavens no," I told him, trying to keep my focus on the test drive.

Thoughts began to blur in my mind a bit as people and things began taking on more abstract meanings. The car I was test driving, for example, symbolized my ability to carry on with my life without limitations. Its brightly waxed red finish practically glowed in my eyes with its promise to take me into a boundless new horizon.

When I told the salesman that I had no way of producing the fifteen hundred dollars he would need to give me the car, I could see the disappointment in his eyes. I left the car lot, realizing that no magic carpet would whisk me away from my troubles. The promising aura surrounding the car lot faded into the distance as I continued to contemplate, on foot, what action to take.

I had to make my way back to Huntsville in order to work at the Holiday Inn; so for the first time in my life, I rode on a Greyhound bus. At the bus station there was an African American man, in what appeared to be a security officer's uniform. In my fuzzy state of mind, he seemed profound, telling the clerk that he had done some "detection work" the previous day about one thing or another.

The discussion that I was listening to seemed to take on some greater relevance to me as my mind began swirling. As I sat in the bus station waiting for my ride home, I began connecting one seemingly random detail to another, about a great many things. One concept linked with another in a pattern that left me continuing to ask myself more questions. After connecting an endless array of dots, I took my seat on the bus to begin my journey home. It was at this exact moment that my second psychotic break with reality hit with full force.

One moment I was sitting in the bus riding back to Huntsville on a sunny day, thinking at a fast pace and connecting concepts, and in the next moment I could feel my mind twinge and vibrate, collapsing into a deep level of psychosis. At that instant, I felt like I was on another plane of existence, and I could read people's minds—again.

The amazing thing was that it never occurred to me that I had been through all of this type of thinking before. All of the sudden, it all made sense and Bert had been right the whole time. He wasn't delusional at all, but filled with the most exquisite manner of divine truth. While my application to law school was at an end, a period of six weeks in a severe state of psychosis was only beginning.

HOTEL COUNTER AT THE EDGE OF TIME

I returned to Huntsville on the bus from Tuscaloosa in a highly delusional state. Bert was still living with us; except now, instead of me trying to convince him that his ideas stemmed from a mental illness, we were very much on the same page, in terms of the delusions we were experiencing. In fact, I was learning from him new ways of interpreting the distorted input my mind received. The clinical term for this phenomenon is folie a deux, but I would not learn this until many years later.

The way Bert described how he interpreted his surroundings was that every building he walked into was a mansion that he owned due to spiritual power. I came to believe that I was a powerful being touched by God, as well, and that I had ownership of far more than my station as a desk clerk at the Holiday Inn implied. Bert helped me to see that I had possessed this type of power the whole time, but was only now becoming aware of it.

I clocked in for my shift at the Holiday Inn, as always, only this was now an experience much grander than the hundreds of times I had done so before. This time, I thought that I, in fact, owned the Holiday Inn, if not the entire world that the hotel inhabited.

On the first day of the job in this psychotic state, I walked over to the counter at which I worked thinking that I was a part of the family that owned the hotel. Thoughts of Mafia figures, who I thought owned things like hotels, pervaded my mind as I strutted behind the desk.

While I know this is not in accordance with the enhanced level of spirituality I alluded to earlier, it is the nature of psychosis as one's train of thought shifts rapidly from one concept to the next. The green colors that decorated the lobby shone brightly as my perception was glazed by symptoms of my illness.

I was not at the counter for more than a couple of hours before it occurred to me that there was no reason for me to remain behind the counter at all, since I owned everything, anyway. I left my post and began to walk to the mall that was just a couple hundred feet away. I walked through the mall thinking how awesome it was that I had these wonderful powers and could command so much richness from the world.

I walked over to a cell phone sales booth and talked to a man about buying one. This was the first time I had ever spoken to anyone at the many cell phone sales booths that were so prolific at shopping malls at the time.

The young man at the booth looked at me as if I did not quite belong there, but ran a credit check on me anyway to see if I would be eligible to purchase a phone. It did not take long for him to pronounce that I had awful credit that would in no way allow me to buy a phone. I left the sales booth with my ideas about owning everything somewhat diminished, but my delusions of grandeur continued, as I realized that my ability to utilize my new powers would require a bit of tweaking.

I walked around the mall in amazement for a time, thinking about the marvelous nature of the mall and, of course, my untapped powers. I decided to walk back to my counter at the Holiday Inn, and as soon as I arrived an angry front desk manager confronted me, demanding to know where I had been for the past two hours. Nedra was the woman who had hired me for the job and who was now upset with my behavior.

I told her I had gone to the mall, fully expecting her to understand that this was my right, as the owner of the hotel. She then asked in an exasperated tone, why I had decided to go to the mall. This confrontation seemed very much at odds with my concept that I owned everything and was accountable to no one, and the only answer I had for her was that I simply did not know why I had gone there.

She then looked at the tie I was wearing, which was part of the front desk uniform. The tie I had on had the Kroger logo on it. I picked this tie when I dressed for work that day because I thought that it was a particularly potent token of power, as Kroger had been the first job I had when I turned sixteen years old.

This was the first time I had ever been in any real trouble at my job, and I was again caught completely off guard when she asked me why in the world I was wearing it. I had no good answer to this question, as I did not expect anyone to question why I did the things I did. Nedra asked me to go home and to take a couple of days off work, as I clearly was not feeling well. I took her advice and did just that, not understanding why the things which made perfect sense to me did not seem understandable to her.

Taking a few days off, I did what most people do, particularly when they do not have a car. I watched television. This time, however, when I watched television I thought that the people on the screen could actually see and hear me just as well as I could see and hear them. This phenomenon started out in a subtle way. At first, I became convinced that the two women on a local cooking show were aware of me.

Their close proximity to me, geographically, made this possibility more likely in my mind. The two women on the show, who were the picture of gentility, were not speaking to me directly all the time; most of the time, they would speak to me through subtle innuendos, which I would then have to interpret. Their comments about the consistency of a potato soup for instance, might mean that I needed to become more consistent about my daily exercise regimen.

I also interpreted much of what they were saying to have sexual overtones. These interpretations were very disconcerting in that they signaled that even my most private thoughts were on display for these people communicating with me through the television waves. These ideas, like all delusions, came to snowball in time and grow in intensity. If these cooking show ladies could read my thoughts, then so could the lady who delivered the evening paper, or anyone else. When one believes that other people can read their thoughts, it does not take long to enormously miss the freedom of privacy. It is hard to even imagine a more stressful state of mind to live in.

During this time, I became much attuned to symbolism inherent in both people and objects. I spoke to Bert about this idea at length, and he agreed that he, too, was highly aware of how people and objects were representative of many things. We spoke at length of the appreciation we had for the people in our lives that had provided so much for us. Our grandmother and stepfather were at the forefront of our minds in this regard, and we decided to show our stepfather just how much he meant to us.

We decided to pile up many objects that we felt symbolized the gifts that he had provided us. We gathered toys, books, and all manner of material, and placed them outside the door of his house for him to view. At the very top of this heap of symbolic objects, I placed the paper I had written for my application to law school.

In retrospect, I realize that this action probably caused my stepfather much unnecessary grief and worry. However, at the time, it all seemed perfectly natural to us.

I also gathered together all of the comic books I had collected during my youth and over the last year, when I developed a renewed interest in reading them. Bert and I loaded these objects into his car, and we disposed of them in the dumpster at the church I attended. I did this because my delusions made me believe that these books symbolized concepts of worldliness that God did not want me to contemplate. My act of disposing of these books in the church dumpster symbolized my desire to be rid of ungodly things.

My grandmother later chastised me for this act of cleansing more severely than I expected her to. She found the deed reminiscent of burning books, which was an act she found particularly repugnant.

“That’s like something the Nazis would do,” she said with a sickened scowl.

When I returned to work after a few days, I could see powerful symbolism in everything. The chastening I’d received because of my unsanctioned desertion of the front desk made me realize that I clearly had certain protocols I had to maintain in order to remain at work without upsetting other people. While I checked people in and out of the hotel, they began to take on enhanced meanings. By the end of the night, the people I checked into the hotel were somehow angels, and the credit cards they used were their passkeys to enter this dimension of reality. The hotel counter became a magical gateway by which beings of immense power could navigate their way to our world. Why these beings from a higher plane of existence wished to inhabit our level of reality was not my concern. My job was to make them as comfortable in their transition as I could. I beamed a smile at the man in the dress jacket with no tie when he presented me a gold card, shining with spiritual energy. He had curly brown locks that would rival any archangel. And when he left the hotel counter to enter the inner confines of the dimensional portal masking itself as a hotel, he strode with powerful elegance.

With a cascade of symbolic thoughts reeling through my head, many in different directions, a woman I had been working with that night approached me. She was a black woman who was currently living with her parents and her young child. She had confided in me weeks earlier that she had recently struggled with a decision to have an abortion. Her parents would not have approved. In my usual frame of mind, not distorted by psychosis, I had clearly understood that this was a lady faced with a very human decision about her future and that of her family. In my delusional state of mind, however, her presence seemed to signify something much more sinister.

I left the hotel counter, which was the focal point of so much power, to try to sort out the conflicting concepts battling in my mind. I had to get away from everyone—somewhere—so more answers to this infinite mystery could fall into place. I wandered around the hotel and eventually made my way to the hotel restaurant. It was dark and unoccupied.

Thoughts about the Garden of Eden and the enormous symbolism inherent in that tale came to the forefront of my consciousness. Weighty matters on a universal scale were trying to resolve themselves as I sensed God instructing me to sit down at a table with a booth. I did so, and He told me to close my eyes, lay my head down on the table, and not move until he wanted me to do so. I was very afraid by this time and did as God instructed me to do. I was there for an indeterminable period of time when all of a sudden, I heard a noise beside me.

The woman working with me who was struggling with the potential abortion had searched for wherever I had vanished to and found me sitting in the restaurant with my head down on the table. Her arrival heightened my fear exponentially as I heard her calling out to me.

"Jim, what are you doing in here?"

I thought that I had been transported spiritually to the Garden of Eden, and that she had been some kind of demon sent there to tempt me to open my eyes and defy God's command. I kept my eyes closed and my head bowed, even as she touched my shoulder and whispered in my ears. I could visualize the room in my mind very clearly, and I could visualize her, although her image was distorted into something wicked.

Later that night another lady who was working the night shift after mine appeared and tried to talk me into snapping out of my trance. In my mind, she was another demon trying to tempt me, and I refused to open my eyes or utter a sound.

Hours passed. I refused to open my eyes while my mind remained absorbed in trying to make sense of the mysteries around me. Finally, even Bert appeared and tried to convince me to snap out of my apparent coma. This was a complete surprise! I knew that the real Bert would never collaborate with the demons. One of the evil creatures must have been masking their voice to sound like him.

Eventually, an ambulance arrived, and I could hear the paramedics as they tried to rouse me. Were these more demons trying to convince me to break God's command to be silent? By this time, I could sense the sunlight through my eyelids and could tell it was daylight outside. When I refused to speak to them, they began the laborious task of dragging the muscled bulk of my body out of the building.

They held something that smelled very pungent up to my nose, and I gagged reflexively, thinking about the vinegar held up to Jesus during his crucifixion.

"He's gagging, so he can't be unconscious," one of the paramedics said with a tone of consternation.

Apparently, they had been wondering whether I was actually unconscious or just refusing to move. I could hear them talking to Bert, but I could not make out exactly what they were saying. Somehow, Bert talked them into letting him take me home instead of them taking me to the hospital.

In retrospect, it seemed odd that he did not want me to go to the hospital after witnessing this ordeal, and that the ambulance personnel agreed with him that I should not be taken to the hospital. It turned out that Bert did not want me to have to incur hospital bills such as the ones that I had accrued prior to this incident; and apparently, the ambulance technicians did not want me to do so, either. The end result of this bargain was that the psychosis continued unabated, without the assistance proper medical care could have provided.

I was stuffed into my brother's Maxima, still refusing to open my eyes, or utter a sound. I was now convinced that the ambulance techs were some kind of torturers working for the demons. I thought that they were going to torture me as the centurions had Jesus, as evidenced by the vinegar they had placed under my nose. When Bert drove me away, I thought that he had been allowed to rescue me from the torture, and that I had been rewarded for my refusal to break faith and open my eyes.

I kept my eyes closed as Bert drove mile after mile. After perhaps twenty minutes, I could sense the car parking. I felt Bert's touch as he placed his hand on my arm. In that moment, my eyes snapped open as if his touch had prompted them to against my will.

My eyes were open only for a split second, but in that time, I saw something more terrifying than anything else I have ever seen or imagined. It looked as if I was staring at a vista of hell itself, replete with lava and showers of fire blazing out of control. My eyes snapped shut just as quickly as they had opened, and I felt horrified by what I had just witnessed. Some time after this, I felt the presence of God telling me that it was okay to open my eyes again. I prepared myself to open my eyes, frightened by the realization that I might do so only to rediscover the horrible plane of reality I had just experienced. Ready to snap them shut again, if need be, I opened my eyes. But what I saw was not hell, at all. Instead, it was a parking lot of an apartment complex I had never seen before. The morning sun was cascading serenely through the peaceful clouds above the brown apartment buildings.

"Where are we?" I asked.

"I used to live in these apartments," Bert answered. "Man, am I glad you snapped out of whatever kind of trance you were in. Those guys wanted to take you to the hospital."

"Where are we going now?"

"Back to Grandmother's house, I guess," he shrugged.

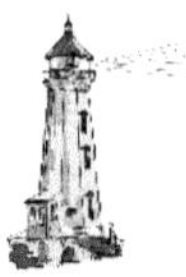

METAPHYSICAL ROMP

With no car and now no job, since my manager told me over the phone that she did not know when I could return to work, I was effectively stranded at my grandmother's house with Bert. I remained in a severely psychotic state of mind, and my notion that the television was speaking directly to me deepened to a level that rendered me unable to watch much television at all without sensing a barrage of messages directed at my psyche. This perceived lack of privacy added fuel to the fire of feelings of desperation, since the law school application seemed to have been my best and final hope for escaping confinement.

Two constants persisted throughout this period of psychotic stress: the need to walk, and the renewed interest in religion. These two drives combined especially well with one another, particularly since I no longer had a car. On a Sunday morning, I decided it would be a good idea to walk to church. I did not walk to the church at which I was a member since it was five miles away. Instead, I walked to Mayfair, a church that was only one mile away on the same street, Whitesburg Drive, which connected to my grandmother's townhouse. Whitesburg Drive held the distinction of being home to more churches than any other street in town.

Twickenham, the church where I held membership, had split in 1979 from Mayfair. I had never been to Mayfair before. There was much talk in religious circles, even outside of the churches of Christ, about the split between these two congregations. From what I could gather, no one actually remembered why the two congregations had gone their separate ways.

In any event, I felt called upon to attend The Mayfair Church of

Christ, and so I dressed in my Sunday suit and hiked my way down Whitesburg Drive as cars whizzed past me.

I arrived at the church very early in the morning; so early in fact, I was asked to help serve the Sunday communion for the people who could not attend the later church service. As early communion ended and the worship service approached, I was surprised to see a number of people from my childhood who had apparently decided it would be a good idea to renew their membership at the church they had originally left. I thought that perhaps the divisions between the two churches had not been as serious as people had supposed. I sat down with an elderly couple to begin the day's worship service. The church was full of people. I had heard that for years there had been plans to move into a new building, and there was barely enough space here to contain the crowd of people. I thought that the congregation might have split apart simply because attendees did not want to be around so many people at one time.

The worship service began in its usual way and proceeded normally up to the time that I began hearing God's direct commands. I was instructed to walk up to the front of the church through the middle isle, in the midst of that throng of people, and then back down the side aisle and out the door. I was not doing this because I thought God wanted me to admonish the congregation in any way; I just did it because I thought that was what He wanted me to do for reasons known only to Him. Never one to question God's direct commands, I followed His instructions, without deviation. It caused much more of a stir than I thought it would, because when I reached the outside of the building two men in suits approached me.

"What's the matter? Are you upset?" they asked.

"No, nothing is the matter; I just have to leave," I said.

I began to walk away from the church. However, instead of walking in the direction that would take me back to my grandmother's townhouse, I began to head in the opposite direction. The parents of childhood friends, the Perkins, lived not much more than a mile from there, atop a hill in an upscale section of town. It was not long before I was reliving the climbs I had made as a young boy, up the wooded steep. I knocked on the door of their house, not knowing what to say to them exactly, but they didn't answer since they were probably in church.

I began wandering through the neighborhood, not really knowing exactly where I should go. I walked past Tommy's parents' house and eventually out of the neighborhood. I cannot remember if it was on this walk or one similar to it that I walked over to my adopted brother, Bill's parents' house.

My mind was really humming in that way it does when it is trying to process large quantities of inconsequential information.

It started raining while I was walking. Bill's parents, Betty and Wayne, could immediately see that I didn't look well, and that it had made no sense for me to walk that far in the rain. They had never seen me in a psychotic state of mind and I told them that I was really zoning out. My feet were hurting from so much walking. They lived at least five miles away from my grandmother's house.

Bill's father, Wayne, wrapped a blanket around my shoulders and said he was taking me to the hospital. Wayne drove me to Huntsville Hospital and waited with me while I went through triage, waiting to be screened for admission. Those are very long waiting periods. It is asking a lot to have someone wait with you in that purgatory of uncertainty. I am quite certain he had other things he would rather be doing on a Sunday afternoon, yet he remained with me for several hours until I was assessed and admitted.

I only remained in the hospital for a few days before I was released. My adopted brothers David and Bill came by to visit me there, and they were quite concerned that the hospital was prepared to release me without ensuring that my psychotic symptoms were under control.

Their frustration with the situation was magnified after they talked to me in my room for a few minutes where I confided to them I was actually a member of the F.B.I. This was one among the many delusions that had been coursing through my mind before and during my hospital stay. The hospital kept me there for one extra day after listening to David and Bill's protestations, and then I was released back to my grandmother's house once more.

Little did I know that David and Bill would soon learn enough about the mental health system to ensure that I would be hospitalized for an appropriate period of time. But before their plans could fall into place, my journey into the unknown world of psychosis would continue unimpeded.

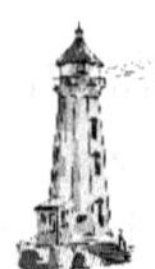

THE LONG RIDE

Nearing the early spring of 1998, Bert and I embarked upon a fantastic voyage of shared psychotic experience. This journey took actual shape with a road trip we made to Alabama's state capitol, Montgomery, and then to the tiny town of Selma. I had read a flier somewhere that a conference was to be held in Montgomery related to minorities and social welfare. Though I had no business attending this conference, in my psychotic state I felt like I absolutely had to go.

While this was a gathering that likely piqued my interest more fully than it did my brother's, he did agree to drive his Maxima for the trip. In a normal frame of mind, the venture would have been something that I would have found fulfilling. In the midst of a psychotic break from reality, the excursion held more of the flavor of a spiritual odyssey.

As we cruised away from Huntsville down the interstate, every color seemed far more vibrant, even though it was a cloudy day. Scenery that in other circumstances would have appeared dim now seemed to emanate a kind of bright light. A bird flew across our path and it appeared to be moving in slow motion. It seemed as if I was able to perceive the bird's motions in extra detail.

The weather seemed to change as often as the shifting tide of my thoughts. It would be sunny for a while and then the sky would rapidly fill with clouds. As we traveled across Alabama's green hills and fields, I had the sense that we were traveling through dimensions of time and space.

My mind wandered to the rolling hills of Scotland, which I felt were somehow connected to these fields in an extra-dimensional way. My thoughts were very much influenced by the woman that I had been in love with, named July, who had stopped answering my telephone calls once I told her that I had been diagnosed with schizophrenia. Her family was of Scottish ancestry and they made their home in the rural South Alabama fields through which we were traveling.

We entered Montgomery, the Alabama State capitol, looking for the conference I had read about with no real need for a reason as to why I should go. We stopped at one of the buildings connected with social welfare and entered in an effort to find out more about the conference. As we walked around the building, I saw that one of the office doors displayed a plaque that proclaimed "Welfare Fraud Investigation" in golden letters. It made me wonder if some punishing angel must inhabit the office in human form.

After asking around about the conference we were introduced by a secretary to a black woman dressed in business attire. She told us that the conference had taken place earlier. We were too late. At that point, since we had no other agenda in town, we began exploring monuments and state buildings.

The sun began shining, and somewhere along the way I ended up with an umbrella that I had taken from the doorway of one of the buildings we explored. I remembered an adage a professor once told me: "People discard umbrellas all the time and another person picks one up, in a sort of mutual exchange." That umbrella seemed to be, by all rights, mine. I began to feel somewhat nervous about it later, when I realized that I had stolen someone else's umbrella. However, this thought was overpowered by the feeling of magic, of exploring the grounds surrounding the state's capitol.

I traipsed across the beautiful greenery with my brother with a feeling of awe. I was not just seeing Alabama's state capital—I was seeing some focal point that connected the spiritual realm to us and our journey. At some point, it dawned on me that we should drive to Selma and see the famous Edmund Pettus Bridge that was celebrated as a historic landmark for the Civil Rights Movement of the 1960's. Civil Rights activists had tried to march across the bridge and were met with tear gas and billy clubs. In time, they were able to cross the bridge, and they ushered in the dawn of a new era of American equality. My feeling of euphoria soared when Bert agreed to continue the adventure to Selma.

Every song that played on the car radio seemed to be speaking directly to us as we trucked through what seemed a tunnel-like road on the final leg of the journey to Selma. The shimmering darkness that now pervaded the sky seemed magnified in an intense way. My mind felt permeated by some kind of dark field that emanated into my peripheral vision, while my direct line of sight, which was fixed on the road, saw primarily the light that somehow seemed much brighter. The song that drifted through the speakers and seemed to touch my very being was "If you don't Know me by Now" by Percy Sledge.

I interpreted this to be an intense manifestation of God's presence, which meant that my brother, holding the wheel beside me, was actually Jesus, Himself. This was a kind of a breaking point for me in the sense that my psychosis had magnified to an intense level due to the extraordinary amount of sensory input my mind had already absorbed.

A bridge is a magnificent structure. The design of the grey metal turrets transposed across a grey sky, which work delicately in unison to support stupendous amounts of weight, would be a marvel to all who had not traveled across one before. The fact that this bridge who so many had sacrificed so much to eventually cross, this bridge who I felt God's Son Himself had led me to, seemed marvelous beyond comparison. In my state of mind, it seemed quite literally to be a bridge linking my own corporeal existence to spaces far more sublime.

I walked across the Edmund Pettus Bridge awaiting some miraculous event or revelation to occur. None seemed to be taking place, so I thought God wanted me to look underneath the bridge. What I saw underneath the bridge, where it connected to the ground, was graffiti written in some illegible script in red paint on concrete. My sense of awe at having made contact with this supernatural bridge was dampened by the realization that I was not receiving some divine revelation. Not knowing what to do, I began walking through the town and was soon separated from my brother.

I walked up to an old country store where several older black men were congregating. I must have appeared rather bizarre to them, since I was clearly wandering haphazardly around town; however, I was surprised to see that one of them, wearing a trucker's cap and overalls, seemed to have some kind of answer for me at last.

He handed me a copy of *The Watchtower* magazine, published by the Jehovah's Witnesses. While I did not realize what this publication was at the time, I felt satisfied to have some token of spiritual power to carry away with me from this journey. And while I never became involved with this denomination, in later years, I would come to know people of that faith.

I left the old store and the downtown area completely and began wandering in residential neighborhoods. I remember seeing small houses that were bright blue and yellow that seemed to shimmer in the grey afternoon sky. At one point, I wandered to a nursing home, and felt it was God's desire that I go inside. I walked in and wandered down the corridors, looking for answers to the ultimate questions. The place seemed drab, despite the effects of my hyperextended awareness, and I do not remember seeing much of the staff, and those I saw didn't seem to take any special notice of me. I looked into one of the rooms and saw an ancient black woman. She was in a wheelchair, dressed in a gown, and she had long white hair. We made brief eye contact, but it seemed to last an interminable amount of time. Perhaps this woman reminded me of my own elderly grandmother who I loved so very much. Whatever the connection, I soon decided that I had fulfilled the directive that had brought me there, and felt it was time for me to leave. Once outside, I realized that I was lost. I had no idea where I could find my brother.

I wandered back to the downtown area and couldn't find Bert. In fact, there didn't seem to be any people about town. I was astonished then to see my brother walking down some sidewalk steps toward me. He said that he had been looking for me all over town. To me, it was as if my prayers had been answered. We both decided that it was time to leave Selma.

Somewhere along the line, I had seen another flier advertising that one of my favorite bands was playing in Tuscaloosa, Alabama. The band was comprised of middle-aged black men who played a collage of oldies hits. I was convinced that should be the next part of our adventure.

On the long trip back to Huntsville, the weather was sunny again, and my hyperextended senses had subsided quite a bit. I tried to convince Bert to drive to Tuscaloosa to see the band, since I had no other means of getting there. I failed. By the time we returned to my grandmother's townhouse, I had talked Bert into taking me to the Greyhound bus station so I could continue my journey alone. I didn't even go inside my grandmother's townhouse.

To someone experiencing psychosis, a bus station seems a

profound place. I imagine that this is a universal principle of all people who experience psychosis, unless perhaps they have been to a bus station on a number of other occasions.

It felt, to me, like an oasis of motion in an otherwise inert world. At the bus station in Huntsville, the lights seemed an especially bright yellow inside and everything seemed pristine and orderly. This was offset by the fact that the streets surrounding the bus station appeared particularly dark and maze-like.

The bus first had to stop in Birmingham before it could continue on to Tuscaloosa. The other passengers on were mostly black, which in my mind confirmed that I was making the right decision in taking this journey. I had, after all, immersed myself that day in a spiritual experience by seeing the Edmund Pettus Bridge.

The whole bus concept conjured up many thoughts of past civil rights struggles. Thoughts of Rosa Parks, who played a key role in the Montgomery bus boycott, as well as the Freedom Riders who attempted to ride in an integrated bus through Alabama and other Southern states, were prominent in my mind. By the time our bus left Huntsville, the effects that the psychosis was having on my brain were becoming more tangible. My brain felt like it was pulsating and then buckling from the strain of processing all of the sensory input.

I kept a bottle of medicine in my pockets, as well as a butterfly knife. It seemed like a good idea at this time to take my medication, which was at the time an antipsychotic called Risperdal. I was certainly not in the habit of taking medication at any time other than when I was in the hospital, but that feeling of physical discomfort inside my skull prompted me to swallow one of the tablets, anyway. It was not long after, because of the effects of the medicine and the mental state I was in, that images began to blur. As I lay back across the bus seat, I stared at the silhouette of a teenage black woman who was facing the front of the bus. Her head seemed to morph and contort in all manner of curious ways as I became increasingly drowsy.

Most people don't realize that antipsychotic medication doesn't typically work instantly. It must build up in one's system over time to have the desired beneficial effect. Tired of seeing the world in this contorted way, I decided to close my eyes; and eventually, I began to sleep. I awoke shortly after we had completed the first leg of our journey and arrived at the Birmingham bus station.

I demonstrated the one trick I knew on the butterfly knife to a person I met after debarking from the bus. The black man in his fifties who drove the bus walked past me, seeming little impressed with my display. The outside of the bus station in Birmingham seemed rather austere, much like the one in Huntsville, but larger. The inside of the station seemed much larger, darker, and somehow more sinister than the station in Huntsville.

It was several hours before the next and final leg of the bus ride began. This was definitely ruining my timetable to be in Tuscaloosa by 10 p.m. It must have been around 11 p.m. when I began to wander around the downtown Birmingham area.

Surrounded by the tall, old buildings, I walked to a large bank that had a wonderful glass storefront. It was a crystalline wall emanating an emerald light. I peered into the bank and saw counters and desks like any other bank, except these were surrounded by that green shining brightness.

I walked through a park that featured beautiful benches and trees that had vibrant red leaves. By this time, I realized that I needed to head back in order to catch the bus again, but I was now hopelessly lost. I wandered around and found myself in a more industrial section of the city. Factories and other fenced off buildings filled the landscape. The streets were devoid of people.

I ran into a solitary black man who was heavy set, wearing a dingy tee shirt and jeans.

"Do you have any pills?" he asked me in a friendly tone.

All I had was the bottle of Risperdal that I had been carrying with me on my journey.

"This is an antipsychotic medication. You can't get high off this," I explained.

He looked at the bottle and shrugged, saying with a smile, "I'll take one off your hands anyway."

I gave him one of the pills, happy that he seemed pleased by the gesture.

After much circling and vexation, I somehow managed to make my way back to the downtown area. I still however, could not find the bus station. At this time, a man drove up to me in what was an older model

Cadillac. He asked if I needed a ride and I told him I was just trying to find the bus station. He said he'd give me a ride. The inside of the Cadillac had a rather ominous feel. I vaguely remember him asking me if I wanted to make some money, which I declined rather bluntly. I did thank him wholeheartedly, however, when he dropped me off at the bus station.

The trip to Tuscaloosa was uneventful. I slept. The bus driver woke me to tell me we had arrived at the Tuscaloosa bus stop and it was time for me to get off. His annoyance at having me on the bus didn't waver; I realized that I was the last passenger on his bus.

When I stepped off of the bus, I didn't find the third bus station, which I had imagined would be there. Instead, I found myself on the side of a strange street and hopelessly lost. By this time, it was early dawn and well past last night's ten o'clock show. My sister and brother-in-law had moved back to Huntsville soon after I graduated and I no longer had any close associations in town. I did the only thing I could think to do: I began to walk. My feet would be very sore by the time I stopped.

My delusions at this point were not at the same level of intensity they had been before. While I continued to perceive a vague sense of beauty in the things I saw, the portentous events and emotional sights I had seen the day before vanished into my subconscious.

My primary focus now was on the fact that I was lost and did not have a destination. I walked around for the entire day, having no idea where I was but continuing my quest to find some point of reference. Thoughts about why I was there and what I would do if I found what I was looking for didn't surface as they would have had I been in a more coherent frame of mind. I simply had to find my way out of the maze and somehow rest my pained feet.

On the first part of this journey, I walked around various neighborhoods and somehow came across a wondrous park that I had never seen. It seemed to contain statues of druids, as well as beautiful shrubbery. Tuscaloosa is known as the Druid City, and there is a park on the campus that has small statues of druids. This was a different park altogether, and seemed to be something of a labyrinth. My memory is sketchy about this part of the journey. Perhaps my mind was so overextended by the previous day's events that my psychosis reached a new apex, where it was the journey itself that became all-consuming and not so much the sights I saw.

I also remember walking down a long stretch of road, once again thinking that my feet were very sore and that I had many more miles to travel. This was a road I had been on before and was somewhat familiar with, because I had even ridden my bicycle down this road when I was preparing for the bicycle trip I made across the country. Yet still I had difficulty finding my way to a place I knew better. At one point, I passed an out-of-the-way club I had frequented as a student of the university, but still could not make out exactly where I was.

I also walked into Tuscaloosa's main public library and paced down the long rows of books, desperately trying to recapture the image of how the location of the library fit in with my other memories of places in the town. By the time I found myself on the more familiar ground of the campus, it was evening. I believe this was sometime in February; however, the weather was unseasonably warm. The simple pair of jeans and button-down shirt I wore were sufficient.

Now that I knew where I was, my mind was able to focus on my consideration of what I should do. The trudging journey to find my way out of the chaotic unknown instead became a stroll down memory lane, determining answers to existential questions, such as, "what was my place in the universe and how did I fit in with God's plan?" Then all of a sudden I realized what my ultimate point of reference should be!

The law school, which I associated with order and the universal good, was the destination I had been seeking the whole time! I limped there, grateful with the knowledge that my journey had not been in vain. The UASL was open and filled with students and staff. I had never been to the law school at five o'clock on a Thursday night and was surprised by the number of people there. I didn't know exactly where to go now that I had arrived, so I walked past beautiful furniture and art décor, discovering sections of the law school that I had never seen before.

Then, I found myself in the law library. I had been in this section of the building before, but not often. When I had worked there several years before, I had helped to make Xerox copies of books, which the school bookstore would then sell to the students. It was rare, then, that my work carried me to a library of books I was not helping to construct. There were a couple of carts of books being given away at the checkout counter, where I asked the librarian if I could have a book on federal law and they said yes. I looked around for a while and left, feeling a renewed sense of vigor.

With my point of reference firmly established, I left the UASL to continue my stroll down the byways of the past I associated with the campus.

It had rained while I was in the law school building and the night seemed somehow illumined more than usual, by a kind of purple blue light. I think one can accurately describe being in a state of psychosis as a feeling of, at times, traveling through other dimensions. Once again, the dimensions I seemed to be traveling through were intimately connected to my past.

Puddles of rainwater brought about recollections of a woman from Minnesota I had dated in college who was one of the great loves of my early life. The large puddles, which seemed to resonate with a luminescence of their own now, seemed to be the Great Lakes of Minnesota, which I had heard about. I felt joy at traipsing across the lakes as if I were some Paul Bunyan-type goliath. I experienced a deluge of other psychosis-fueled imaginings during this time, but this is the instance that stands out most in my memory.

An all-encompassing sense of weariness rushed back over me and my prime point of reference, the law school, soon began to draw me back like a powerful magnet.

When I entered the UASL, again I was not seeking a source of inspiration so much as place to rest my throbbing feet. I happened upon a student lounge that seemed to appear as a magic oasis and stretched out to rest. Law students entered and left the lounge at different times while I propped up my legs, which had now stiffened into pillars of pain. I was primarily focused on getting some sleep. This became less and less likely, since my mind continued to race from one fleeting concept to the next, at an alarming rate.

I continued to wonder what God would reveal to me next, as my blistered feet throbbed. I slept until about ten o'clock at night when I was awakened by what appeared to be a sheriff with a wide brimmed hat and a brown uniform. I wondered at the symbolic nature present in the person. He was most certainly a representative of the law and order that had made the UASL my focal point to begin with; however, he also struck within me a sense of fear with the way he questioned me, and with his no-nonsense attitude. Perhaps this was some sort of angel of death, come to impart clues for the next part of my journey. The truth, of course, was far more mundane than that, and soon this man escorted me to the hospital.

I spent the night at The Druid City Hospital, and Bill, now living in Birmingham, drove to Tuscaloosa and said he was driving me back to Huntsville. On the way out of the hospital, the sheriff with the wide-brimmed hat, who had found me the night before, stopped me. He told me rather bluntly that I was not to come to Tuscaloosa again unless I had some sort of official business there. This was a difficult admonition to hear, as Tuscaloosa had been home for many years. However, I must admit that it had a powerful effect, and I have never gone back unless I have had some sort of business there.

On the ride back to Huntsville, Bill said that everyone was worried, and that they were afraid I might have gone to New York or another random destination. I was stirred by a vague sense of guilt, but I remained fairly silent, as I didn't know exactly how to explain to him what was going on. I cannot recall if he drove me to the hospital in Huntsville, where I stayed for a few days or if he took me back to grandmother's house. The last three and a half days had been just the beginning of a psychotic break from reality that would last for six weeks.

CLANGING CRASH

The television continued to speak directly to me with an ever-increasing deluge of messages that correlated with whatever delusions I was experiencing and sending them in new directions. In my bedroom, I watched a rerun of the Taxi television series from the early eighties, and the television seemed like a dark bubble of life from another dimension. It was somehow allowing the characters to communicate directly across time and reality. The characters seemed to morph, however, into more sinister entities than the characters everyone else knew. Danny De Vito's character exuded a cynicism far beyond the two-dimensional experience of watching standard television. Even the friendly character named John seemed to be the butt of a monstrously incomprehensible joke.

It was as if the television set was a window into another realm, except it was really an open window and the other realm seemed to be able to push out of the bounds of the television screen and into my own reality. Characters on television were speaking directly to whatever I happened to be thinking about and then commenting upon my delusional responses. An ancient shaman staring into a campfire for several days could not create a similar effect, even if he tried. The television set was not a campfire exactly, but it was certainly sending me messages that were causing my mind to careen in previously unexplored directions.

I decided to simply keep the television turned off. How wonderful it would have been if turning off my delusions were as simple as turning off the television. Unfortunately, it was not, and my psychosis continued, whether or not I was tuned into the television. It began to seem as if the television could see what I was doing, even when it was off. The ancient shaman can always stop staring into the fire when he knows he has finally had enough. I was not allowed that luxury while experiencing psychotic symptoms. I could not stop the delusions that people were watching me.

In my mind, I was in the mafia, working for the government, and some kind of religious figure all wrapped up in one. Even if I did not know the exact details of the role I played in the grand scheme of things, I felt I was rapidly gaining clues into my own significance to their design. Bert didn't help the situation. He said he knew exactly what I meant when I described this confusion to him. He described certain people in our lives to be avatars or symbols of beings of great power. My grandmother, for instance—who was eighty-two at that time—was like a deity, and Bert brought her offerings in the form of trays of food. In his mind, it was not the food itself, but the act of kindness that satisfied her hunger.

When contemplating this the next day, Bert's theory seemed to make a great deal of sense. It was as if I could feel her power and desire to be loved emanating all the way from her room downstairs. She was not a person, in the general sense of the word, but indeed a being of great power, with no real need for a physical form.

In the early months of 1998 it was expected that the United States might begin a bombing campaign of Iraq at any moment. News coverage of this crisis was broadcast constantly, and people were rather uncertain about whether or not we would soon begin a second war with them.

Continuous coverage of the impending event, broadcast over my television, took on a decidedly ominous aspect. Since the television was speaking directly to me, the dramatic nature of events was exacerbated. While I had been avoiding television as much as possible, I have always been an avid current-events junky, as well as someone very interested in the fate of our nation. I found myself unable to resist the lure of witnessing what would happen next. As my symptoms persisted, this great crisis, unfolding across the land that was once ancient Babylon, grew beyond geopolitical proportions to biblical, and I became an active participant, as well as a viewer.

The United States needed to view my eye movements and reactions to what they were showing on the television in order to plan their strategy for what to do next. This was because I had so much psychic and spiritual power that a special government agency had selected me for their project. I could read the minds of Iraqi leadership like a medium, and this agency could read and interpret my reactions in order to understand what the Iraqi army would do next.

The news anchors, who were informed by the government of what was going on, indicated this to me through subtle gestures and innuendo. When I moved my eyes, they moved theirs in ways which seemed to beckon me to provide more of my input. I felt it was my duty to continue to watch the broadcasts into the night, so that the government could monitor my reactions in every detail. This was why I had been the focus of such interest, via television waves, the whole time. My mind continued to strain at the cascade of images from the television screen combined with delusional thoughts, which connected everything to something else.

The next morning, after having experienced being the government's guinea pig, I was no better off, in terms of understanding what was going on in the realm of reality. My grandmother left her bedroom upstairs and walked down the staircase in order to sit down in the living room for a while. This was something that she did only rarely these days, since it was very difficult for her to get around. She sat smiling in one of her antique wooden armchairs as she read the newspaper with a magnifying glass. Her eyesight was continuing to fade every year. I no longer saw her as something other than a person, however. Now I saw her as someone who could offer me divine guidance.

The nature of psychosis is such that delusions change shape often, as the mind strains to discern each new reality. Grandmother told me that there had been a great mudslide in town, on land that was once owned by my grandfather. This disaster was on all the local news stations at that time. My grandfather, who was my grandmother's first husband, had been a wealthy landowner, and had apparently sold land that was prone to the types of mudslides she was reading about to build houses for a subdivision.

I felt it was my duty to somehow restore the family honor which had been besmirched by this disaster, but I didn't know how. Later that morning, after my grandmother had gone back upstairs, I was divinely inspired about what I should do next. My firearms had been returned to me by my stepfather since I had not had a relapse of psychotic symptoms in close to a year and a half.

I was to take one of my rifles and walk from my grandmother's house to the site of the mudslide. This would remedy the problem in some supernatural fashion, of which I was not yet aware. I was not to load the rifle, as this was to be an act of symbolism designed to heal old hurts and not one intended to cause fresh harm. Somewhere in the back of my mind, I also realized that it was legal in Alabama to walk around with a firearm that was not loaded, or I thought that it was, anyway. Any delusion I ever experienced was also tempered by the knowledge that I did not want to go to jail. Perhaps it was this basic understanding, as much as anything, which prevented me from doing anything illegal during my psychotic breaks with reality. I had, after all, studied the law intensely in an effort to be admitted to law school.

Many people with mental illnesses end up behind bars for petty crimes. I learned many years later that it was common practice, before behavioral health medicine was used in local hospitals, to arrest one for a petty crime before he could be committed, simply because there was nowhere to house them while they were in a mental state that warranted hospitalization.

I was extremely lucky that I had an understanding of the law, and that I was born in a time and place that prevented me from becoming one of those unfortunate people whose legal histories follow them throughout their lives.

I now knew what I had to do. However, with war fever over Iraq clouding my vision, I couldn't make up my mind about which weapon would be the most appropriate to carry. I narrowed my choices down to an assault rifle, which was the Egyptian version of the AK-47, and my grandfather's shotgun. I decided to seek my grandmother's guidance in deciding which one to carry on my righteous quest.

I did not ask her this question directly, because I assumed she parceled out wisdom in the same symbolic jargon as the anchors on nightly news. I handed her the breakfast that Bert prepared for her that morning and she asked for a fork. I decided to base my decision on which weapon to carry determined by which fork she chose to eat her breakfast. Did she want the long fork, which would represent the

Egyptian war rifle, or did she want the short fork, which would represent the shotgun? She said, with a smile, that she preferred the short fork, and so I went downstairs to retrieve the formal looking short fork she instructed me to get. I was now armed with the knowledge of which token of powerful symbolism to carry with me in my endeavor.

Shotgun in hand, I left the house and began walking, with only a slight notion about where the mudslide had actually occurred. The streets were ominously quiet as I walked through the neighborhood surrounding my grandmother's townhouse, the shotgun slung against my shoulder, like a good soldier. No one seemed to notice me at all as I carried my magic shotgun through the neighborhood. I crossed a major thoroughfare into a neighborhood with grander houses. Militaristic visions of glory bombarded my mind as I walked through the quiet streets. Thoughts about my family and its honor and what it meant to this city swelled in my conscious mind.

I began thinking— nervously at this point, as the reality of the situation began to surface a bit—about my cousin, Bill, who had been an important part of my life from age seven to age twelve. He had been a fighter pilot in World War II and retired as a lieutenant colonel from the United States Air Force.

"Your grandfather was good to me as a child, and now I intend to be good to you," he told me, after meeting me while I was living with neighbors shortly following my mother's death.

My grandfather had been a self-made man who, like Bill, had grown up in a poor rural community.

From the day we met, Bill brought me with him to church on Sunday and Wednesday and took me fishing in a boat on Guntersville Lake at least twice a month. He was able to answer every question that a child with an inquisitive mind might ask. He taught me about everything from the birds and the bees to the history of the United States. We never seemed to tire of one another's company, and he became one of the defining figures of my formative years.

"A good parent doesn't care if their child likes them or not," he told me once. "The parent's job is simply to raise the child in a proper fashion, regardless."

His passing when I was twelve years old, like my mother's passing, would be a loss more fully understood only with the passage of time.

In my psychotic frame of mind, while marching through the streets, he suddenly began speaking to me directly, telling me not to be afraid and telling me in which direction to walk.

I walked by expensive looking houses with well-manicured lawns. It was Sunday morning and there was hardly anyone outside. I began walking closer to the main thoroughfare, Whitesburg Drive, as my cousin Bill's voice instructed. Eventually I ran into a familiar building from my past. I was at the Elks Lodge!

My grandmother had a free lifetime membership to the Elks Lodge, and my grandfather had been a member there in its heyday, as well. My grandmother had taken me there every Friday night when I was a small boy, where we would dine on savory fried catfish and I would drink Shirley Temples. We would watch *The Incredible Hulk* on the television. I still remember the sad piano music that would play during the credits while Bill Bixby walked in the rain with his knapsack slung over his shoulder. The club had a darkened atmosphere that only enhanced the shimmers of light that the television cast on plate and glass.

Now, as I marched past the Elks Lodge, shotgun in hand, I recalled visiting the club a couple of times in the past year without Grandmother, courtesy of her lifetime membership card. Grandmother had quit attending the club for the last fifteen years, saying that the club stirred up too many bad memories.

Seeing the Elks Lodge amplified my thoughts about family pride. My cousin Bill's voice now mingled with the voices of my mother and my ancestors whom I had never met before, including my grandfather, to become one commanding throng of voices.

These ancestral voices said that it was now time to walk back down the main thoroughfare toward Grandmother's house, carrying the shotgun. I had to overcome my fear in order to do so, because somewhere inside I realized I might be making something of a spectacle of myself. I never did discover exactly where the landslide had occurred; although, I am sure it was some number of miles away. The voices, however, told me to have courage and to complete my task as instructed, despite the modification in plans. I made it across several blocks of the main thoroughfare, with cars zooming past me, when something startling occurred.

In my peripheral vision, I saw a police car pulling up next to the sidewalk. In the next instant, I was staring at the muzzle of the most brightly polished silver pistol I could have ever imagined, held by the black-mustached policeman driving the car. In the instant after that, I could hear the loud click of the giant gun as it was being cocked, as it continued to be pointed at me.

It is a very frightening and indeed sobering experience to be looking down the barrel of a handgun. The voices subsided to a degree in that instant, enough for me to do exactly what the voice holding the gun ordered me to do, and that was to place the gun I was carrying down, and to put my hands behind my back. The sobering voice holding the gun then began asking me what I was doing as its owner began cuffing my hands behind my back. It did not take the police officer long to determine that the gun I had been holding was not loaded, and as I had thought before I had set out on this adventure, I had not committed a crime. Another police officer joined him, and unfortunately this police officer was one with which I had a history.

One night, many months before, I had been carousing at a popular nightclub, which had I walked to since I had no car. I had become quite drunk and had called a cab to take me home. The cab driver became upset over something I said or the fact that I had no money, or some combination of the two, and refused to give me a ride home. At that point, I decided to simply walk home, since I only lived two to three miles away.

Walking through downtown Huntsville was a different experience in the middle of the night, and while intoxicated. I had no fear of walking at night. After all, I had walked through downtown Memphis, which was much larger and reputed to be more dangerous than Huntsville, and had not been bothered.

This time was different, though. I made it past the downtown area and started walking through a series of neighborhoods, bringing me without incident into the neighborhood where I lived. I finally made it to the large thoroughfare which I needed to cross in order to enter my neighborhood. As I crossed this lighted thoroughfare to enter the seemingly pleasant darkness of familiar streets, something that seemed out of this world occurred.

A group of young white toughs, too many even to count, rushed me from out of the dark. There were so many of them and it was so sudden that it seemed they were actually falling out of the surrounding trees. One of them gave me a light punch to the face and they had me on the ground in no time, screaming for me to give them my wallet, which they simply took without my help. The wallet only contained a few dollars, which was the main reason why I was walking home in the first place. They threw the wallet at me. Now, completely broke and feeling so much like rubbish, I stumbled my way to a drugstore a block away and told the clerk what had happened. The story sounded bizarre even to my ears as I explained it. I lived in what I thought was a reasonably nice neighborhood, after all. I had certainly never heard any tales of this kind occurring in the area before, and apparently, the store clerk hadn't either.

I asked the clerk to call the police, and as soon as the officer arrived on the scene it became immediately apparent, to my stunned surprise, that he was hostile toward me. I was still somewhat under the influence, and the police officer apparently thought that the story sounded about as incredulous as it had sounded when I had described it to the clerk.

The officer then began questioning me thoroughly, and in a manner that signaled to me that he thought I was probably contemptible. I became upset with his attitude since I had, after all, just been the victim of a violent crime, and I let him know it in as much of an outraged tone of voice as I was willing to display to a police officer.

This soon escalated to a point where the police officer called for backup. The new police officer had a smoother demeanor, even if he seemed to share his partner's distrust of me. He asked me to empty pockets and I obliged him, grudgingly. What he discovered caused him to raise an eyebrow in suspicion.

It was an ordinary tobacco pipe. I was not even smoking cigarettes regularly at this time. However, I had picked up the habit of smoking tobacco out of a pipe from an elderly and wise friend who I had hung out with at one of the bars I frequented. Although I thought it looked rather cool and different, it now caused me no small amount of frustration as I tried to explain to the officer that I had the pipe merely for the purpose of smoking tobacco.

Although I think he believed it to be the truth after much sniffing of the pipe, he did not really support me in any other way or take very seriously my complaints against the other accusing officer. In the end, they would not even drive me the rest of the way to my house. I had to walk home alone and afraid.

The police officer now joining the officer who had ended my psychotic trek with the shotgun was the one who had initially answered my call following my mugging. All the memories of the prior encounter began bubbling to the surface as the gruffness of the recent arrival's voice barking out questions barraged my psyche further.

At this point, something even more surprising occurred. Bert pulled up in his beat up Maxima, and got out as quick as a rabbit to try to see what was happening. Looking as bedraggled as usual, he said some words to them that I could not really overhear, and amazingly, he convinced the officers to remove my handcuffs and to let me go home with him.

As I walked to my brother's car, however, the officer who I'd had the past experience with asked me a question that I cannot remember. But the answer I yelled back to him as I entered my brother's car remains something easy for me to recall.

I told him emphatically, "It's because you're a jerk!" He'd give me his answer to that later, but at the time, it seemed to go unchallenged.

Bert drove me back to my grandmother's place.

When I arrived home, I remained actively psychotic. I spoke on the telephone a couple of days later with my adopted brother David, a man who had visited me at the hospital numerous times. He had heard about the incident involving the police somehow, and began questioning me about it. He asked what had happened, and I explained to him, "Grandma, said that I should do it."

"That certainly doesn't sound like something that she would ask of you," he said.

I then explained to him how Grandmother had communicated her wishes to me based on the type of fork she chose to go with her breakfast, fully expecting him to grasp this concept as something that was perfectly rational.

"I'm sure that is not what she was trying to tell you," he said.

"Oh, I see," was my reply.

His explanation did jar me back into reality to some degree, and I understood that what I had done was clearly misinterpreted by everyone.

"I'll talk to you later on," he said.

I watched a mobster movie and began to think I was a reincarnation of the historical crime figure, Lucky Luciano. When Bill telephoned, the conversation led at one point to me explaining to him how I had recently wiped out on a bicycle going downhill at high speed. I actually did an entire flip, and this accident could have killed me or caused me severe bodily injury.

When I told Bill that I had walked away from the accident unscathed, I said to him, "Well, you know that they call me Lucky, right?"

No one, in fact, had ever called me Lucky, in either my memory, or indeed the memory of anyone that knew me; nor did any of the wide range of nicknames I had collected over the years denote any implication of luck. I was met by a stunned silence after making my pronouncement, and this was the first time I had ever known him to be at a loss for words.

Another idea that crept into my mind, as I watched cable television, was that the female therapist I had seen for some time previously was in fact a sexual surrogate that would be willing to help me to overcome my sexual inexperience. With this in mind, as well as with the glimmer of real insight that the HMCMHC could help in a more practical manner, I decided to make a trip there just as soon as I possibly could.

On Monday, I did just that, making the mile long trek from my grandmother's townhouse to the HMCMHC, dressed up in a sports jacket and slacks. When I arrived, I was informed that my therapist, Marilyn, was off that day, but that another therapist, Mary Beth, agreed to meet with me for a short time in her place. She had bright, intelligent eyes and short blonde hair.

Mary Beth undoubtedly had little trouble seeing the glazed look in my eyes, and scheduled me to see my previous therapist in the very near future. Memory of this period is somewhat hazy; however, what I believe happened next was that when I returned for my scheduled appointment, a pair of sheriff's deputies met me. In no time, they had me in custody and whisked me away to Huntsville Hospital. They informed me that someone in my family had filed a petition for a hearing to determine if I would be committed to a state hospital. Until that hearing, I had to remain at Huntsville Hospital. The hearing was to take place in about a week.

This was all very new to me, because I had never been in any kind of legal custody before. I later learned that this was quite a common practice with people who suffered from serious mental illness. I was grateful for the fact that I already had dress clothes on hand. I spoke to my stepfather and let him know what was happening and discovered that he felt very strongly that I allow his lawyer to represent me at the hearing. He thought that would give me the best chance of not being committed. I certainly didn't want to be committed, since I had absolutely no idea what that entailed. Druid City and Huntsville Hospital had not been that bad, but I had only my grim imagination as a template for what it might be like to reside in a state mental institution. My stepfather sent his lawyer, who was probably in her late fifties or early sixties. She had short grey hair, and a stern look that signified the fact that she had been a female attorney in times when most attorneys were men.

She asked me if I wanted her to represent me at the hearing or if I preferred to have my court-appointed lawyer represent me in the case. She said this in a tone that seemed to indicate that she had no real desire to influence the decision one way or another. I had met the man who was appointed to represent me, and he seemed competent.

Some intuition I had told me to go with the court-appointed lawyer instead of my stepfather's friend. Not wanting to see my stepfather's money at risk of going to waste motivated my decision.

I knew the probate judge hearing the case, as he had actually presided over my grandmother's petition to adopt me when I was sixteen.

Before I would make a second appearance in front of this judge, however, I first had to stay in the hospital and undergo an assessment from a mental health professional who would determine if I was someone who would benefit from state hospitalization. I felt compelled to truthfully answer the man who assessed me, even telling him about thinking that my therapist was a sexual surrogate.

At the hospital, I played games that a pretty woman in her early twenties facilitated. Trembling with embarrassment at the situation, I threw bean bags at a stationary target in front of her. She, like other pretty women my age who staffed the hospitals, was brutally aware that

I was confined there because of symptoms of a mental illness.

By the end of the week, I was still delusional, and readied myself for the big hearing. I think that it happened to fall on Saint Patrick's Day, and I garbed myself in the dress clothes that I had on hand for the occasion. I believe the jacket was tweed, and it was a coat that I never really wore at all. I had searched through my closet to find it before my walk to the HMCMHC. Of course, I made sure that I had on green for that day.

When I entered the small, wood-paneled courtroom where the hearing was to be conducted, I noticed a number of my family members. My adopted brother David was there. It turned out that he was the person who had filed a petition for my commitment to the state hospital. In order for a person to be committed, someone must file a petition with the appellate court in that county. Bert, surprisingly, was there as well, looking not only as bedraggled as always, but also unusually nervous.

The probate judge asked all witnesses to swear or affirm that they would tell the truth, the whole truth, and nothing but the truth, so help them God. Then they all began describing the gory details of my situation, in alarming detail. My attorney informed me that I should not testify under any circumstances unless called to do so, and I knew that a person should always heed his lawyer's advice. However, I was unable to resist speaking out when I heard the police officer say something that was not accurate.

The police officer said that when I left the scene after carrying the shotgun, I told his fellow officer to go to hell. The judge swore me in, despite my attorneys' quiet urgings not to testify and his eventual sigh as he resigned himself to the fact that I would. I pronounced to the court that I would affirm the truth. My religious upbringing came to the forefront then, as I had remembered reading in the Bible that it was sinful to swear to anything aside from your own word. I told the court that I had said nothing of the sort as it related to what the officer just swore to, but that I had, in fact, called the officer a jerk.

A broad smile creased the officer's face, and I could hear snickers from the spectators in the tiny courtroom. I had just seriously damaged my case. The judge read his ruling, which consisted of unintelligible legal jargon. I looked over at my attorney to try to figure out what it all meant, though I only remember him wishing me luck in the sincerest tone he had managed since I first met him. Then I was whisked away by sheriff's deputies to the garage, located somewhere in the darkened bowels of the courthouse, and then into their car, where I was ushered into the backseat.

Looking through the mesh screen, separating me from the sheriff's deputies in the front, I asked them where we were headed.

"We're taking you to the state hospital, in Decatur," one said.

"Ah," I said.

I noticed a toothpick on the floorboard and wondered why my focus was so fixed on its delicate form.

WAY STATION

My level of fear rose exponentially with each mile in back of the sheriff's car. I had no idea what was in store for me, and I wondered if the state hospital would be like prison, or even worse.

My overactive imagination, as well as the memory of the prison flicks I had been fond of watching over the years were my only guides for what this institution might be like. My delusional state continued, although to a lesser degree than before, since I had been consistently taking antipsychotic medications for a week.

With my imagination running away like a freight train, I went into the mode of someone who was getting ready to be processed into a prison. In other words, I was ready to fight or do anything I needed to do to keep from becoming assaulted or abused while there, even if this meant I had to start getting into fights right away or start crafting shanks out of flatware.

After a thirty-five-minute drive, I was driven up what was affectionately termed "The Hill" to one of the state mental institutions. It was housed in an extremely old three-story building and was surrounded by trees and other vegetation. An iron sign at the bottom of the hill read "North Alabama Regional Hospital" (NARH).

The fear of being in a prison was exacerbated, at this stage, by staff members that weighed me and took me to a shower. A delousing agent was provided, and the way they barked out orders lent itself ominously to the idea that I was being put in a maximum-security institution where unimaginable dangers lurked in every corner. While I was in the shower, a large black man with a wild tangle of hair was taking a shower in an adjacent stall. My feelings of trepidation were heightened as he began singing the song "That's the sound of the men working on the chain gaa-a-ng." Not knowing what else to do, I began singing the song along with him, as we showered in our separate stalls.

After showering, I was walked down a long hallway and shown to my room, where I was introduced to a man who I was told was to be my roommate. In his early sixties and politely mannered, he was getting ready to go home any day. He told me that he lived in a rural community. I would never have known that this man had ever had a mental illness if not for the fact that he was sharing a bedroom with me in a state mental institution. We got along quite well, and I had no fear of sleeping in the same room with him.

The room was Spartan; it had a chest of drawers, two closets, and two single beds. The windows had bars on them. These served as good reminders to everyone in the facility that their freedom to walk among people in mainstream society had been revoked for as long as the state deemed necessary.

It didn't take me long to make the initial discovery that the environment I had to move about in would at first be one that was rather cramped and restricted. I was in level one, which meant I had highly restricted freedom to move about the hospital grounds.

The next day, I found there was a sitting room, which was about twenty by twenty feet, my bedroom, and a small room filled with crossword puzzles and board games. This was the extent of my physical world. People in my status would have to "level up" with good behavior in order to have full freedom of movement within the hospital.

I met a few of the other patients on my floor and felt a strong rapport with most of them. I began to relax my guard a bit and we played board games until it was time for lights out at ten o'clock. I awoke early the next morning to discover a large hospital orderly standing over me. He insisted that it was now time to get out of bed. He demonstrated the proper way to make a bed, which he insisted that I do repeatedly until he was able to bounce a quarter on it.

Until I leveled up, I would have to dwell in the sitting room for hours on end, since we weren't allowed to simply lie in our beds, except for a thirty-minute nap after lunch. There was an older television set without cable in the sitting room, which was full of people. They were mostly people who stayed at level one for one reason or another. People with higher levels tended to spend time in other parts of the hospital grounds. Most of the people in the sitting room were older than me and many of them were extremely symptomatic, in terms of their mental illness. Someone might start screaming or crying at one of the hallucinations or delusions they were experiencing at any time. Many of them simply talked to themselves for long periods of time.

I had to exercise a form of mental discipline that allowed me to endure the noise of the sitting room. I had to tell my mind to try to focus on whatever television program was on instead of my chaotic surroundings.

Every couple of hours or so, we would get a smoke break where we would ride an ancient elevator up to a terrace enclosed in a mesh screen. There was an assortment of snack machines and Coke machines there. My grandmother ensured that I had pocket money to spend while institutionalized.

The smoke breaks were an important part of our daily routine, in terms of socialization and getting a break from the enclosed surroundings of the hospital walls. I was not a regular smoker when I entered the hospital, but I did smoke an occasional cigarette. People offered me cigarettes during the smoke breaks, and I found myself smoking much more frequently than before. As a result of this experience, I became a regular smoker for many years afterward.

I discovered also that the hospital had some stimulating entertainment, especially after patients moved up from level one to level two and finally to level three. There was a pool table and large—what are now considered old-fashioned—videogame machines.

There was also a popcorn machine in a room where a popcorn social was held on my second night in the hospital. I remember getting into some sort of argument with the large orderly who showed me how to make my bed. My hand, trembling with rage while holding the paper popcorn bag, spilled kernels of its precious contents on the floor. I cannot remember what the argument was about, exactly; I only remember that I managed to regain my composure. It is important to note that I was still delusional at this point, thinking that I was all sorts of things, including a mafia Don or the reincarnation of various people, such as Elvis Presley.

I soon found that people began looking up to me for leadership and guidance. I'd never been considered a leader in any other time or setting, and had usually found myself being the equivalent of the class clown in various social situations.

The realization of this interesting new role became clear one night in particular, as my group of friends hung out on the terrace during a smoke break. The hospital was divided into two main floors, and on this night, both of our floors had a smoke break at the same time.

Still in a moderately delusional state, I felt drawn toward a young man of East Indian descent from the other floor, who I could tell, through his grace and demeanor, was the leader of the people on his floor of the hospital. I walked up to the man and shook his hand, introducing myself. He seemed to shimmer with a sort of personal magnetism which drew other people toward him.

He introduced himself to me and said, “I can see that you have a lot of spiritual power.”

I was surprised to see that he was looking at me with the same admiration in his eyes with which I had gazed at him. In the frame of mind I was in, I saw this as some sort of monumental meeting between two beings of great significance. I could even feel the cosmic power streaming through the beams of the hospital and into me, and my new friend, as I looked on his smiling face, illuminated by the yellow lamps lighting the terrace. This was the first time in my life that someone who appeared amazing to me had looked at me with such a sheer look of appreciation.

Smoke breaks were not the only times of critical importance to me and the other patients at NARH. Mealtimes were also an escape from the monotonous floundering around the confines of the institution. I found the food at the hospital to be quite tasty, and it was rumored that Morrison’s Cafeteria Company also catered the hospital cafeteria. The eggs were clearly powdered, but I discovered that I didn’t mind the taste. We gathered in the dining room in orderly groups, determined by the staff, of thirty people at a time and received our trays, cafeteria style. We sat down to enjoy our meal at round tables which sat six people. Although I never pocketed any forks for making a shank—there were no knives—I will admit that the thought ran through my mind from time to time, particularly on occasions when I would have to stand up to one bully or another. These oppressors were not as pervasive as they surely must be in prison; however, they did surface from time to time.

There was one incident early on, when I was assigned a new roommate who was clearly delusional. He went on and on about how he was in the Mafia and was not someone to be trifled with. In my own mental state, I was a mafia figure as well, along with so many other things, mostly religious, and I could hold my own against anyone. He was from my hometown of Huntsville, and that was eventually where we found common ground and a way to lessen the friction between us.

Another focal point of the hospital was the pay telephone that people waited in line to use. I would sit in that dark wooden booth that someone had built by hand, like a confessional, and attempt to reach out to people I cared about and who I thought could offer me guidance through this life-altering experience. My grandmother had given me a phone card to use only in case of emergency. I soon ran up a large tab on it, though, as I felt the need to reach out to anyone who could comfort me in this dark time in my life. I spoke mostly to my grandmother, who provided her usual share of comfort and wisdom in these conversations.

I had the recurring thought that it must really be breaking the heart of a person who had already witnessed more tragedy than most people can dream of, to have to be living through another of her children's battles with mental illness. In thinking about how she could endure such tragedy in her life, I think back to some of the things she often told me over the years. Many times, I heard her make the remark, "I have traveled the world, you know." She had been to Europe, Japan and a number of other places few Americans, especially of her generation, have had an opportunity to visit.

I think that she realized that this statement would hit home with me one day. I think that she was trying to say to me that she'd had the opportunity to live a fulfilled life. I think that she held on to memories of all of the people she had helped, as well as the other meaningful experiences which fueled a lifetime as rich as hers. Maybe, this was her challenge to my future self. Could I utilize the advantages she had helped provide me to live a rewarding life?

Easily, the most emotionally painful conversation that I had in that telephone booth was the one I had with one of the women I had dated off and on throughout college, whom I will call Katy. She had been a tennis player at the University and had left that sport to pursue sorority life.

Katy was from Minnesota, and her beautiful blond hair and blue eyes lit up my nights in Tuscaloosa like the Aurora Borealis. A few months prior to my current hospitalization, I had reestablished contact with Katy after having lost contact with her following my first hospitalization in 1996. We had spoken together on the telephone a number of times since then. I decided not to let her know about my diagnosis at that time. The nightmarish situation that had followed me telling another of my old girlfriends about my diagnosis, when I never heard from her again, guided my decision making process in this matter as much as anything else.

I decided to give Katy a call on the payphone at the state hospital and let her know everything. I felt like I needed a friend more than ever at this low point in my life. When I told her that I had schizophrenia and was now in the state hospital, she was alarmed. Her voice quavered.

"You're really scaring me!" she said.

She hung up.

Many years in the future, something called a smart phone will become commonplace, and most people will interact through something called social media. Katy and I will renew an acquaintanceship in this way and even speak on the phone again twenty-two years from this moment. Of course, I have no way to know any of this while in NARH in 1998.

I cannot help but notice recently that the media, in commercials on television, encourages people not to end friendships with another person just because they are diagnosed with a mental illness. I wish those kinds of commercials had been broadcast when I was in my early twenties, and I can only hope that people heed the words of these ads today, so that some other young person may not experience the same degree of rejection that I felt that day simply because I had a medical condition.

Instead of speaking to a beautiful young woman in the hopes of a blooming romance, I was now in a locked-down universe, where another beautiful—and older—lady was interviewing me for an entirely different purpose. She was the hospital psychologist who gave me an assessment and decided what classes I would take during my stay.

All patients had to take classes that focused on coping with mental illness. In these classes, I learned even more about the other people who were patients. They were of all ages, backgrounds, and diagnoses. It did not take me long to see that I had much more in common with these people than I had differences, as we all talked about ways to prevent finding ourselves back in the hospital.

After a week in the facility, the staff determined I was not a serious flight risk, and I was promoted to level two, where I had considerably more freedom to move about. The best part about this privilege was that it allowed me to escape the psyche-smashing monotony of the sitting room. There, Bonanza continually played on the television, and I had to endure the continual sounds and actions of people who, in many cases, had lost control. I found that the library was a good place to go, especially when I didn't feel like being around other people. There was a radio in the room, and I enjoyed searching the dial for soothing music, and listening to sounds from the early eighties.

I had not thought much about my deceased mother in the past, but when I listened to that radio and heard those songs from my youth, I thought a great deal about her and the fact that she had been a patient in this same hospital more than once.

Many times it felt like she was even speaking comforting words to me through the radio, and I couldn't stop myself from weeping. I found myself reconnected to her in a way that I had not felt since the time of her death in 1982. Our shared experience of being confined within the walls of this same institution bonded my mother and me in a profound way.

After two weeks at NARH continuing to take regular dosages of psychotropic medication, I completely phased out of the delusional universe that had consumed me. The greatest change to my thought processes was an internal monologue that occurred while I was still delusional.

"I am surrounded by people, most of whom are all describing the same ideas that I have, and there is no conceivable way that we can all be right. Another man claims to be Elvis, and therefore, we cannot both be Elvis. That man claims to be in the Mafia. That idea sounds absurd, except for the fact that I myself have the exact same idea about myself. Therefore, it must be equally absurd that I am a mafia figure."

This logic helped me considerably to break out of the psychotic state I had been in, to one degree or another, for the past two months.

It is important to understand that logic, in and of itself, is not enough to break out of delusional thinking, because reasoning can often be circular. Being around so many other people who had a mental illness was a good remedy, though, and the state hospital was the perfect place for me to get back on track mentally.

There was a man about my age who had a very agreeable personality. He was admitted to the hospital at about the same time as I was, and he tended to be in my circle of friends. He was in a delusional state for a period longer than mine, and he described to me the delusions of grandeur he was experiencing.

I found myself trying to convince him that his delusions were, in fact, just that—delusions. I did that by using the same form of reasoning that had helped me to find release from my own psychotic state.

"Ten different people are saying that they are Elvis. How is it possible that they are all correct?" I would say.

Although he was not convinced at first, it didn't take many days of my careful coaxing, combined with his heavy regimen of antipsychotic medication, for him to reach a state of reasoned thinking. He felt quite awkward and embarrassed about the delusions he had suffered a few days earlier, and about him trying to convince me that they were real, but I comforted him by explaining that there was nothing to feel embarrassed about, since we were all in the hospital because of similar episodes.

That experience marked a very important turning point in my life.

First: I would never again experience psychoses that approached the magnitude of the earlier breakdowns. My illness continued to affect my brain and my life in various other ways. But losing all control of my faculties due to my psychotic disorder was something I would never endure again.

Second: I discovered that I could be successful in reaching out to and working with other people who had experienced mental illness. While this talent took a considerable amount of time to come to full fruition, the notion that it existed came into being precisely at this time. In this sense, my confinement at NARH was an opportunity for growth, and certainly was not the frightening experience I thought that it might be when I first entered its mysterious walls.

HOME FIELD

With my return to reality, there came an increased desire to get out of the state hospital. There was, as well, the nagging question of where I would go once I left. Although I was completely free of psychotic symptoms after the first two weeks of my stay, I stayed in the hospital for another month. While this seemed unnecessary at the time, it was the reality of the situation I faced. While I didn't expect to be one of the rare people who was confined in the hospital for a year, I didn't know if I would be forced to be there for perhaps six months. The fact that I remained confined in this facility whether I was beset by symptoms or not was a sobering lesson in life.

I was encouraged by the fact that I moved up to level three, and now could walk around the grounds of the hospital at my leisure. There were no fences surrounding the facility and nothing to stop me from walking away from the hospital. I knew, however, that no real good could come from leaving. I was happy about this, in one sense, because I could resume walking to exercise as I had been doing for the past year or so.

I had a number of visitors while in the state hospital. Bert dropped in most frequently. Grandmother made sure that he came to see me once a week in order to make sure I had money, underwear, and anything else I might need. My adopted brothers, David and Bill, visited me one time.

David and Bill were in their late twenties, and they talked with relieved glee about the difficult time they had getting me into the state hospital, and how thankful they were when I finally engaged in enough wild activities to end up there. They warned that they could get me back into NARH if they needed to, and if necessary, they would have me committed to Bryce, the state hospital in Tuscaloosa. When they said the word Bryce, they pronounced it in such a way as to indicate that it housed people much worse off than where I was. People tended to say the name of that state hospital with a mixture of both dread and awe, and David and Bill were taking the opportunity to keep the tradition alive, in order to keep me reigned in.

Interestingly, Bryce was considered a state-of-the-art facility when it was built in 1860, and its founder Dr. Bryce was a pioneer of promoting reforms in the treatment of PLMI. The hospital later declined markedly, and became overcrowded and less enlightened with the passage of time. In the 1980's it became more enlightened and less overcrowded again but maintained the same—by now ancient—physical structure, which was historic in its own right, being one of the largest buildings of that design. Following the events of this story, the facility was rebuilt as a beautiful new hospital, featuring all of the latest advancements in mental health care and retaining the name Bryce. Ironically, the name is still used to invoke fear into patients not wanting to enter into a higher level of care who, generally speaking, have no idea that it is an extremely fantastic facility to the point that it is rather luxurious, featuring stimulating game rooms, spacious courtyards with fencing concealed from view, and even a beauty shop.

My adopted sister, Kim, also visited me, and her sorrow at seeing me in these circumstances was clearly visible despite her best efforts to conceal it.

With every year that passes, I become increasingly convinced that this entire situation impacted her and everyone else in my extended family far more than I could have imagined. This is in stark contrast to my increasing understanding that my grandmother was able to handle all of what happened to me with a greater acceptance than I could conceive.

Another heartbreaking visit was from my stepfather, Dave. I sat with Dave on the gigantic steps outside the hospital. The bitter irony that he had visited my mother at this very hospital on several occasions before her death, sixteen years earlier, did not escape my consciousness for a moment. I smiled, though, and did everything I could to convey to Dave that I was in charge, not only of my faculties, but also in charge of my surroundings. I emphasized this point during our conversation. When one of my friends brought me something, or perhaps gave me a message of some kind, it clearly demonstrated to Dave that I was important to that person. Dave did manage to find a smile and began advising me in terms of how I should live my life.

He began asking about the job at the Holiday Inn and what I liked about it. I began to describe the various perks of the job, as well as the responsibilities. He told me that he thought it would be a good idea for me to go back to that job, and that I should try to be satisfied with having a job like that, and it was not necessary for me to fulfill the great ambitions that I had held since childhood.

"It's okay for you not to take on too much stress, Jim," he said.

Dave's sense of understanding could be seen in his smile, and if he was deeply saddened by having to visit me at the same hospital where he had visited my mother, he managed to do an extremely good job of not letting it show too much in his expressions.

He had invested a great deal, both financially and in time, in me, and it must surely have been as difficult for him as it was for any of my family members to see my downward slope into the world of multiple hospitalizations. Somehow, he managed to view me in the same compassionate light that he always had. There is an important lesson for all family members to learn from people who are hospitalized for having a serious mental illness: This does not have to be the end of the world, or your relationship with the person who is ill. Someone can be hospitalized for having a serious mental illness and eventually go on to live a fulfilled life. A visit to the hospital does not have to be like going to your loved one's funeral.

Another development that took place during my time at NARH was a romantic relationship that brewed between me and another patient. It was not long after I ceased to have psychotic symptoms that I met a woman, who I will call Lorraine, in order to protect her confidentiality. She was probably in her late forties, and she was an attractive woman.

It had been a year and a half since I was first diagnosed with schizophrenia and about three years since I had experienced any kind of serious romantic relationship.

Those three years did not unfold the way I thought they would. I was athletic, intelligent, and I thought I was what most people would consider a physically attractive man. There were many moments after I was initially diagnosed with my mental illness that I longed for a monogamous relationship with someone I could settle down with.

I found out in short order that having a mental illness hampered my prospects in this area even more than I had initially thought it would.

It did not take very long in the limbo of this thought process for me to think about some of the young women that I had no particular desire to date in the past as most desirable prospects, in retrospect.

"Why on earth didn't I try to date her, or her. If only I had tried to settle down with her, or anybody I was involved with, at least I would be in a romantic relationship now." My thoughts ran along.

"I have been completely robbed of that part of my life," I thought.

I was delighted to meet a woman who did not seem to have a problem with my having a mental illness, or with our age difference. We began as friends, but the relationship soon escalated into something more. She told me not long after she met me that I was "smarter than the average bear," and she seemed to find that appealing. She said she had a condition called bipolar disorder, and her daughter had committed her to the state hospital. She also said she was happily divorced.

Lorraine was from Decatur, the town near the hospital, and she was able to tell me a great deal about our surroundings. She said that the crumbling building that we were in was once a hospital for people with tuberculosis and that this was the reason why I was given a T.B. test when I was first admitted.

The only thing I knew about tuberculosis was that it was what eventually killed Doc Holliday, the legendary gunfighter on the winning side of the O.K. Corral gunfight. I knew it was a very bad way to die, in a time when there was no real way to treat it. From time to time the hospital van took us to restaurants or on other outings. On these occasions she would describe the various scenery we passed. The scenery was completely alien to me.

Lorraine seemed to vibrate an aura of not worrying about what was going to happen in her future, immediate or otherwise. She said that she had been baptized a number of times, in various churches. I thought this was a curious oddity. We enjoyed each other's company, learning a great deal from one another. While I am certain that I got the better end of that part of our relationship, soaking in all of the information she provided, I was confident that she could appreciate the friendship of a kind younger man, including protection from the occasional bully.

I came to learn from Lorraine that symptoms of her bipolar disorder, formerly known as manic depressive disorder, caused her to have manic symptoms which compelled her to do things like spend money she did not have, as well as an inability to sleep that lasted days. She would experience bursts of energy that allowed her to engage in activities she would not normally have the ability to perform when she was not manic. While this aspect of the illness felt incredible to her while it was occurring, the net result was that she would feel extremely depressed when the energy burst was over. I never did discover what she had done to be committed to the state hospital, and for some reason I did not feel a reason to pry too deeply into her immediate past.

In the course of our relationship, within the confines of NARH, we had the opportunity to discuss many things. One recurring theme of these discussions was what we would do once we left the hospital. Lorraine said that she thought that it would be wonderful to become a psychologist of some kind, or to work with PLMI in some other way.

"After all," she asked rhetorically, "who can do a better job helping a person than someone who has experienced the same thing?"

It was not long before I took up this cause as well, and proclaimed that I, too, would like to learn how to become a helping professional for PLMI.

At one point during my hospital stay, I had the opportunity to meet and talk with a person called a peer support specialist, who was a Consumer of Mental Health Services (CMHS), as well as a staff member of the hospital. This black man, who was a few years older than me, let me know that I had individual rights, despite the fact that I had been confined to the state hospital, and he was able to answer a broad range of questions I had about the mental health system, in general. His very presence was also a signal to me that there could definitely be a new life for someone with a mental illness, in terms of helping other people.

In the back of my mind, though, I wondered if I had enough life experience or knew enough about working with people to be effective in such a role. I did not know for certain what would happen with my law school application, which was still being processed. And my stepfather's admonitions about overdoing it were still fresh in my mind. In time, this idea of becoming a helping professional in the world of mental health was filed away in my mind, along with all the other ideas I had of making a future for myself.

My experience at the state hospital also marks a point at which I recognized that I truly did have a mental illness. Living and interacting with so many people, many whom were so similar to me, had the effect of solidifying in my mind that I was not just a victim of unusual circumstances.

I had the opportunity to see the full gamut of PLMI and the full range of symptoms they experienced, and how the experiences they had changed over time. This was convincing evidence to someone with a fundamental belief in the laws of logic and reasoning, that I was not being hospitalized repeatedly due to random chance.

When I could admit to myself that I had a mental illness, it became natural to consider that I was part of a community of other PLMI, as well. No desire I might ever hold in my heart to be a lone wolf, wholly reliant upon himself, would ever negate the fact that I was a part of a group of people, larger than myself.

With the acceptance of my situation solidifying in my mind, I began to talk to Lorraine and my other friends about what their living arrangements would be like when they were released from the hospital.

What I discovered in these discussions was that many people, particularly those who did not have anywhere to move back to, were expecting to be placed by the social worker in some kind of housing situation. These people stirred in my heart the flames of hope that I could find a better living arrangement than the one I had—sharing space with my psychotic brother.

I decided to try to speak to the social worker who would determine where I would go upon my release. I discovered that I had to make an appointment to see her. So after a few days, I talked to my social worker, mustering all my charm in an attempt to make a good impression. She was middle-aged with a thick frame, long blond hair, and wise looking eyes. I described to her some of the things I wanted to accomplish in my future, including law school.

"Inch by inch and life's a cinch; but yard by yard, life's really hard," she told me. "If you can remember that, it will help you to make your way through life."

The truth of her words is impossible to deny; I essentially had to switch to an entirely different mode of doing things or else I would become overwhelmed with trying to achieve too many goals at once.

She also informed me that since I was from Huntsville, she would arrange for me to meet with the representatives of the HMCMHC who visit the state hospital routinely to complete housing placement. She said that I'd meet with them in about two weeks. To say that I was excited about meeting with them is an understatement. The prospect of going back to the living arrangement I had been in was horrifying to me, and the fact was that I, like many others, didn't have anywhere else to go.

While contemplating this reality, it suddenly dawned on me with startling clarity: I had already been offered a place to live, by the HMCMHC!

When I was first diagnosed with my illness about eighteen months ago, or what seemed then like a lifetime ago, my therapist had offered me the opportunity to move into an apartment program operated by the HMCMHC. At the time, I was very afraid of the restrictions that I felt surely would accompany such an arrangement, and I was quite comfortable living with my grandmother. I made this decision at a time before I finished college and before Bert moved into my grandmother's home. At that time, I was fixed in denial about my illness, and the thought of moving into a dwelling for PLMI was not a reality I was prepared to face.

Now that I was clear-minded and able to make good decisions, I began to enjoy the added freedoms at the hospital. I roamed the grounds and made use of the facilities at my leisure. The state hospital had now become a pleasant place to be.

I attended weekly religious services at the hospital, which were held by a black minister who I believe was a Methodist. Not as many residents attended these services as one might expect, but the ones that attended were fervent in their songs and prayers and listened intently to the minister's words.

Lorraine attended church services in the hospital with me on at least one occasion, and she confided to me that she had a flock of her own. I do not mean "flock" in the figurative sense; I mean that she had an actual flock of live sheep living in her yard. She had her own home, in the country, where she lived with her mother. As part of her manic symptoms, she had collected a large assortment of animals over the years, and the flock of sheep was her latest addition.

There was another young man in my group of friends at the hospital who I will call Steve. He spent a lot of time with Lorraine and me. Steve had Cerebral Palsy, as well as a serious mental illness. His palsy was so severe that he practically had to drag one of his legs behind him when he walked. He was diagnosed with the same mental illness that I had, and like me, he was from Huntsville.

Unlike me, he held on to some delusions that he could not shake entirely. He believed that he had been communicating with angels on a regular basis and that this was not only plausible, but also wonderfully true.

In 1998, it was in vogue in the media to talk a great deal about angels and people's ability to communicate with them. Steve was not even willing to entertain the notion that his angels were part of any psychotic symptoms. He felt they were, in fact, the real deal. No matter what techniques I tried to help Steve rid himself of these ideas, they rebounded off deaf ears.

After two more weeks, I was shown to a room inside the hospital where I met the people representing the HMCMHC and their housing program. In my mind, this was like a job interview on steroids, and I really went over the top in my efforts to wow and be polite to the two women who conducted the meeting.

Instead of a job interview, I suppose one would call this a living interview, since they would determine if I would have my own place to live. The women seemed receptive, and as I left the meeting I had the impression that they would go to bat for me. About a week later, the hospital social worker delivered the good news, "You've been approved for the apartment program!"

The feeling of excitement I experienced was tempered by the knowledge that what I was thrilled about was an entirely different vision than what I thought my life would be not so long ago. Nevertheless, I was grateful to know I had somewhere to live, away from Bert.

It was now just a matter of winding down my time at NARH until I embarked upon my new life journey with the HMCMHC. I continued to spend time with Steve and Lorraine, as my group of friends steadily dwindled down to just that pair. I learned that my friend, Steve, had also been approved for the same apartment program and that we would be seeing more of each other whenever we were both released from the hospital.

My experience at NARH taught me that the state hospital in Alabama was not in fact the awful place I imagined it to be, but was instead a place where I enjoyed being, and a place that had allowed me to unlock potentials I barely knew existed.

While I was forced to finally come to terms with the fact that I was living with a serious mental illness, I was actually granted a kind of freedom, with the knowledge that there were institutions in place that had my welfare in mind. While my grandmother and stepfather were very liberal in their outlook, it somehow never penetrated their consciousness that housing programs for people with disabilities existed. Their experiences just didn't allow them to see that to be the reality.

They had both lived through the Great Depression, and they had spoken to me often about how seriously this affected their outlook of the world and society. As stated previously in this work, I was trained to think of the world as a more fearsome place than what my own eyes indicated it to be. In this sense, having been raised by elders from a different generation had advantages and disadvantages different from that of a traditional nuclear family. One advantage was that I expected less from the world and society, and I was disappointed less often. The obvious disadvantage was that, up until this time, I had been terrified of what my future held, in terms of living with a mental illness. Although I continued to be highly uncertain about exactly what my future held, I knew I was getting ready to embark on a new part of my journey through life and, at 23 years old, I had accepted my role in an entirely new sort of family unit.

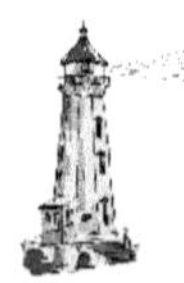

HOMECOMING

My psychiatrist determined in the spring of 1998 that I was ready to be released from the state hospital and return to my hometown of Huntsville. I rode with the HMCMHC staff to my new home there. I had been a patient at NARH for six weeks, and it would take some time to adjust to living in a world that wasn't restricted by bars on windows and the constant presence of uniformed staff.

The Shelter Plus Program had its offices in an apartment complex filled with tan, two-story, wooden buildings. There were apartments scattered throughout the complex for residents of the program. Most of the apartments were rented to the public at large. These apartments were completely indistinguishable from the units housing clients of the HMCMHC.

I lived for my first six weeks in the program in a building containing four apartments set aside for people in the early stages of Shelter Plus. Whenever I graduated from that stage of the program, I would receive my own apartment, which I would be allowed to rent at a cost based on my income. In the beginning phase of the program, I had a roommate and received a number of services designed to help me get my "sea legs," in terms of living independently.

One service included something known as case management. I was assigned a case manager whom I will call Jill. She was a very nice woman, not much older than I, although she was infinitely more knowledgeable about how to adapt to a new environment. It was her job to work on my behalf to ensure I had access to resources that met my basic needs.

One of the first things Jill did was take me grocery shopping. She told me she had access to about forty dollars for me to spend on a one-time grocery shopping excursion, and that I would be responsible for purchasing my own food and items for the house from then on.

We went to Kroger, which also happened to be the same grocery store where my stepfather, legendary for his frugality, shopped. She led me down the aisles, showing me the price stickers on each item, and asked me to calculate the price differences of various products. This may sound like a simple concept, but it opened my eyes to bargain shopping.

I was also expected to attend Day Treatment for four hours a day, five times per week. Day Treatment, at this point, no longer seemed the living nightmare it had when I was first diagnosed with my illness. This was true because I had gained so much experience in being around other PLMI during my stay at the state hospital.

The staff who worked in Day Treatment consisted of people who seemed genuinely interested in our welfare. Fay was the black female therapist—nearing retirement and blessed with an abundance of hard-won knowledge about PLMI. She had a warm smile, which connected her with anyone she met, and a short cut afro hairdo that proclaimed timelessness.

There were two younger people on staff, who were also "getting their feet wet" in the mental health field. One was a young, pony-tailed Hispanic man from New York, named Derrick, and the other was a tall, Caucasian young woman from a rural Alabama community named Meagan. These people were not much older than me, and my pride was wounded because I knew that as their client I could not develop anything other than a professional relationship with them. In a way, this made me feel like an untouchable. I could feel their excitement when they discussed the graduate study they were engaged in. I felt envious, in a sense, that their lives seemed to be moving forward while my dreams were at a standstill.

When I saw my therapist, Marilyn, for an individual appointment, she seemed delighted to speak to me since I was now free of psychotic symptoms. Some of the delusions I experienced during my psychotic break with reality related to thinking she was a sexual surrogate, and I was very ashamed, fearing that she would not want to work with me anymore because of this. This did not affect her connection with me, however, and our therapeutic relationship continued as if none of those delusions had existed.

My mind was now firmly fixed in reality. However, I was soon to discover that my new life would be far different from that of most other people. I would be interacting with a new community of people as I learned to live as independently as I could as a PLMI.

To begin with, my new roommate and I did not get along—at all. One night we had a heated argument about whether or not one had to use hot or cold water when rinsing dishes. Because of our mutual dislike, I avoided him as much as possible. However, I really had no choice as to whom I would be living with. I tended to gravitate toward my neighbors in the building who were also a part of the beginning phase of the Shelter Plus Program.

One woman in the program was in her late fifties or earlier sixties. She had the aristocratic air of the Deep South about her. People were usually shocked when they learned from her that she had lived for many years in New York City as a homeless person. She called herself a "bag lady." I suppose that this did not shock me as much as it would an average citizen of the United States, as, technically, I was considered homeless. I discovered this when my case manager was trying to assist me in receiving some service over the telephone and stated that I was in a program for homeless people. What could hammer home the seriousness of the reality I found myself in more than that?

There was another older woman from the North, who I "clicked with." However, it took much longer to really get to know her than it took with the other members of my new circle of friends. Eventually, we drank many cups of coffee together, talking about our lives and hopes. She cooked stuffed peppers, and I devoured these exotic delicacies with delight.

I became fast friends with a middle-aged African American man, who I will call Ezel. He was a jolly fellow, with a tinge of bitterness over the fact that he had lost his marriage along with a lot of assets and personal belongings when he experienced his first psychotic break with reality.

These three people made it clear that smoking cigarettes was and always would be part of any gathering they attended. My smoking addiction was firmly in place by this time, as I became a full-fledged member of the smoking circle.

My friends smoked constantly, as did my case manager, Jill. She would take drags from a type of thin cigarette that seemed like it would leave a person choking for more nicotine than ever. Her smoking preferences aside, she provided me with enormous assistance in my time of need.

One thing Jill and I had to work on immediately was to take care of the business regarding my disability payments. She drove me to the Social Security Administration (SSA) office and accompanied me as I went in to speak to the staff. They had been sending disability payments of two-hundred dollars a month while I was living with my grandmother. Now I would receive the full payment of five hundred and fifty dollars, thirty percent of which would go toward paying my rent. Grandmother gave me accumulated payments of two hundred dollars, which totaled to about eight hundred dollars. She had been too afraid to spend any of the money, thinking that the SSA would eventually ask for all the money back.

I cannot overstate the intensity of shame I experienced going into the SSA office to ask for disability payments. I felt that I could work as much as anyone else if given an opportunity to work at a job consistent with my level of education. I had lost everything, however, and was now trying to get back on my feet. I thought I would need access to the resources for which I was eligible.

I also applied for food stamps at the Madison County Department of Human Resources (DHR). At that time, an innovation had come on line at DHR; it was the Electronic Benefits Card, which was a kind of credit card with food stamp funds on it, instead of paper stamps. While awaiting the outcome of my disability claim, I received one hundred and twenty dollars in food stamps on my card each month.

While I was adjusting to my new world of food stamps and social security, my friend Tommy had graduated from the school of engineering at the UA and had been hired by a defense contractor in Huntsville. He was living his life's dreams, dating constantly, and making more money than I could even dream of. It was not long after I started living at the Shelter Plus Program that Tommy was buying a brand-new two-story house, in the ritzy outlying suburb of Madison. In his mind, abundant living became the norm, while in my reality, survival depended primarily on not being too proud to accept help.

Although I had regained my basic freedom to move about in society without the restriction of being confined, my freedom of mobility was limited because I still did not have a car. Huntsville had a new bus system, but it took two hours to get anywhere.

PLMI are no more likely to harm others than are people in general. The vast majority of other PLMI that I have met seem even less prone to violence than the average person.

I soon found out, however, that there are exceptions to every rule. My roommate and I did not get along, and as it turned out, my roommate did not get along with many other people, either. One night, after we had been arguing, I was in my bedroom trying to sleep when I heard a lot of rustling outside my door. I told myself to mind my own business and remain in bed. I eventually managed to fall asleep, despite the feelings of nervousness, which kept me awake for a long time.

The next day, I discovered that the man I was rooming with had left the program abruptly in the middle of the night. I thought that this was certainly odd behavior, but I was grateful for the prospect of having the apartment to myself for a while. I cannot remember how much time elapsed between this incident and the time I saw on a news broadcast that this man eventually shot and killed his ex-wife! I felt, in some sense, that I had dodged a bullet, myself, and I made a mental note to be more determined to avoid unnecessary confrontation with people.

I never would have thought that a person with the potential to kill another human being had been living with me in a tiny two-bedroom apartment. I really was living in a strange new world, far different from the one that Tommy and my other college friends were accustomed to.

For two weeks I was alone in the apartment, and then I was told that my new roommate would be Steve, who along with Lorraine, had been my friends at NARH. I'd kept in touch with Lorraine and she was scheduled to be released soon.

Steve moved in and we were both glad to have as a roommate someone we already knew. He fit right in with my new friends, who seemed pleased to have another member under the age of fifty in the group.

After Lorraine was released from NARH, we continued our relationship, though it was now a long-distance one. I relied on her to drive her mother's small pickup truck, which was on its last legs, in order for us to visit one another. She showed me Decatur's charming downtown area, by starlight.

I learned about herding sheep when I helped her round up the animals living in her yard. It didn't take long for me to weary of this activity, though, and Lorraine's mother, who could see that Lorraine and I were more than just friends, now firmly disapproved of our relationship. She found the vast differences in our ages to be absurd and told Loraine as much. Our relationship, like so many other long-distance romances, fizzled and my presence in Decatur ended for a time.

After six weeks, I received the individual apartment I was promised and began furnishing my new place. The Salvation Army supplied a one-time voucher for various furnishings, and I bought some furniture from my adopted brother, David. I was also able to use my antique oak bed from my old bedroom at Grandmother's house.

From the moment I moved into Shelter Plus, I realized on some level that I wanted desperately to be able to move out. My gratitude at having a place to call my own was dulled by a sincere desire to escape my life's circumstances. It did not take much gazing around my surroundings for me to realize that I had, in fact, been in a situation very similar to this one before.

From the age of four to six, I had been taken from my foster parents, along with Bert, from his foster family, to live with my father in the Portland, Oregon area. From age five to age six I had lived in an apartment complex with my father and brother in a lower socioeconomic community. While we were moving into our new home on the second floor of a brown, three-story, wooden apartment building, my brother and I were met by a welcoming committee of neighborhood kids. One of these kids was an African American child named Ray. He was a couple of years older than I was. He asked me something that I was unaccustomed to hearing, and my answer obviously displeased him in some way, or perhaps it was the red hooded sweat jacket I was wearing, because the next thing I remember was being peppered by punches to my face.

This was an entirely new experience, and I was at something of a loss about how to react. At some point, while the punches kept coming and I became increasingly frustrated, with tears streaming down my face, I realized that I was supposed to hit him back. In fact, I could hear

Bert repeatedly yelling at me to hit him back. I sent one punch to his head, which rather stunned and silenced both the crowd and Ray for an instant. After that, Ray began punching me at an even more rapid pace. It was not very long after that when Bert led me away and into our new apartment.

I lived in this apartment complex for approximately ten months, before my brother and I went to spend summer vacation in Huntsville with my mother and my stepfather, where we made up our minds to stay in Alabama with them. Bert made the decision, and I can still remember him telephoning my father to inform him that we were not returning to Oregon. The nine months I lived in the apartment complex with my brother and father in Oregon left a lasting impression on me. Living in that environment activated primitive instincts in me that lie dormant in most people. My survival depended upon being able to find food and avoid angering larger children.

I lived in a household with few groceries, and with a much older and much larger brother who was very upset about the circumstances we found ourselves in. He also had a penchant for taking his frustration out on me.

My father was away from the apartment for much of the time, since he would disappear on "walks" in which he would not be seen for days and sometimes weeks at a time. I learned to find toys by rooting around in dumpsters, since there was no one to supervise me. I learned what it was like to be stigmatized, even by the other poor children around me, who at least had clothes that were clean and that fit them properly. I hardly ever bathed, unless my brother Bert forced me underneath the tub faucet after deciding I smelled too rank.

There was a boy who was about thirteen, Bert's age, who lived upstairs and was deriding me mercilessly one day for my impoverished situation. Bert later explained to me that the boy upstairs was upset because he, too, had fallen from a level of higher economic status into more humble circumstances with everyone else who resided at the apartment complex. The one time my father spanked me was immediately following an encounter with this boy. He was cursing me and spitting on me down the stairwell of his upstairs apartment. I was shouting, crying, and trying to spit back at him only to discover that my own spittle simply fell back on me. My father pulled me into our apartment and punished me for being a part of the spectacle.

I also had the opportunity to learn something about the group dynamics of children in the neighborhood. I remember, vividly, sitting on top of a hill in the school yard next to the apartments when some of the bigger and older children declared to me that I could either come down from atop the hill and join them, or they would come to the top of the hill, and I would be sorry. It did not take me long to leave the hill to join them, although we did not spend a whole lot of time together after that.

The brothers who led this gang wore the same trucker's caps, checkered flannel shirts, and work boots that the children on a small farm in the rural south might wear. One time, I was in their downstairs apartment with them and their parents while they were watching a television show I had never seen before. They had a color television set, by the way, while my family did not. The television show they seemed delighted to watch was the Dukes of Hazard. This was an action show about a family living on a farm in a southern rural community. They spent their time in sports cars, chased by the outlandish sheriff. It was kind of like the Andy Griffith Show on crystal methamphetamine.

I spent then, as I did throughout my childhood, a great deal of time by myself, walking around in my ill-fitting pants and floppy dress shoes, contemplating the world of my inner imaginings. One day, I was walking around the school playground and felt an intense pain in my skull. An instant or so later, I saw the smiling face of Ray and realized that one of his thrown rocks had hit me in the head. Stunned from the sudden ice pick of pain in my skull, I walked in the other direction to avoid further conflict.

Another day, the boy who lived upstairs and with whom I had been involved in the incident for which I was spanked, bullied the wrong person. He picked on one of the children who had convinced me to come down from my hill much the same way he had picked on me. That child had an older cousin, who wore a larger version of the trucker's hat, checkered flannel shirt, and work boots that his younger cousin wore.

He beat the boy upstairs viciously while I stood as a witness, along with the other neighborhood children. A couple of weeks later, I was wandering through the field behind the apartment complex when I looked behind and saw a shape ducking down to hide in the long yellow weeds. When I looked behind me again thirty seconds later, the shape, which was much closer now, would duck back down in the weeds. After a time, I looked behind me to discover the boy from upstairs standing directly behind me. He had been tracking me down like some kind of leopard. I thought I was finished.

"I bet you thought that was pretty funny when that guy beat me up, didn't you?" he asked.

Not knowing how to respond to this query, I merely shrugged.

"I'm going to let you off with a warning this time, but just remember not to ever mess with me," he said.

"Yeh, alright." I quickly agreed. I sighed with relief when he began walking away from me.

Experiences like this taught me a great deal about the laws of human existence; and the chief one was, to be in impoverished environments is to be avoided whenever possible.

Back in Huntsville at the Shelter Plus Program, the backdrop of an impoverished childhood, which I thought I had escaped forever, rushed back up to greet me.

As I walked around the ramshackle neighborhood I was now a part of, I could feel all of the old oppression come back like a tidal wave. As I stepped on bits of crushed glass, which perpetually covered a long-abandoned tennis court in the complex, and through the streets of dilapidated houses and cheap apartments surrounding the neighborhood, I became overwhelmed with the feeling that I might never escape this environment again.

My new neighborhood was only about one square mile. Some strange twist of fate, and of school zone gerrymandering, put an impoverished neighborhood right in the middle of both a lower middle-class neighborhood and into the business section of an upper middle class area. I lived only a couple of miles away from half-million-dollar homes, in a neighborhood with no sidewalks, where practically no one would be brave enough to walk at night.

One side effect of returning to this environment was that I completely stopped the walking exercises I had been so devoted to for the past year. Seeing the shabby neighborhood on foot, I felt depressed and I slipped very rapidly back into being overweight and lethargic. Despite the encouragement by my grandmother and my therapist to maintain a healthy lifestyle, their admonitions took a back seat to my desire to just smoke cigarettes and sit around. Bert was still living in my grandmother's home, and I would visit them both, on occasion.

I am ashamed to say that I had not yet learned my lesson about the importance of taking my antipsychotic medication, despite reproaches from all of the experts, as well as the very profound lessons of my own experience.

Although I had reached a point where I acknowledged that I clearly had a mental illness, I thought that this knowledge and acceptance would be enough to safeguard me from further psychotic symptoms without the need for medication. I figured that if I ever did experience psychotic symptoms again, the knowledge that I had mental illness would "kick in" and I would be able to counter the symptoms with my own will power; or barring that, I would simply begin taking the medicine before the symptoms could escalate.

My experience in the state hospital and in living in my new community had profoundly changed my perspective concerning other PLMI. I did not see them as completely "other" and could accept that we had many similarities. I became friends with the people who lived in my community and learned that, just as in any other community, there were people I could count on and others who would try to take advantage of me.

My friend Steve, whom I had spent so much time with at NARH, would remain my friend for some time, but he was slipping gradually to a place where I did not want to follow. He believed the voices of the angels he constantly experienced were completely real and not related to mental illness. This did not fit well with my experiences, and I became frustrated with fruitlessly trying to argue Steve out of his delusions.

He also smoked marijuana and used other street drugs, which I didn't. I continued to enjoy drinking on occasion, which is certainly something that is unadvisable for one with mental illness, but I knew that using other drugs would be worse for me in just about every conceivable way.

I knew, absolutely, that I had a great number of problems that I didn't know how to cope with, and that I did not need a whole host of others that would accompany drug use. I did not know how to escape my situation and felt certain that it would take a longer period of time than I thought I could handle. I would rather feel depressed and hold on to the few resources I had while trying to change my set of circumstances than to lose everything to the hollow joys of street drugs.

I received my official rejection letter from law school while I was coming home from the Twickenham Church of Christ. An older couple had kindly given me a ride to church and dropped me off at my grandmother's house, after stopping by the mailbox. While I was waiting for a ruling on my disability claim, I also asked the church for help. I received seventy dollars and some food from the pantry. I began feeling awkward about attending church, especially in light of my recent psychotic experiences. Many of these had been religious in nature.

I thought that everyone at the church knew that I had a mental illness, and that I would be rejected because of this difference. I believed that the people at the church probably knew even less about mental illness than I had when I was first diagnosed. To be around so many people who knew that I had a psychotic disorder and who were not a part of the mental health community was not something I felt prepared to handle. I thought that in the future I might find a church to attend where people did not know everything about me.

Before losing heart about attending church I had considered strongly and seriously becoming a minister in the Church of Christ. This possibility had been in my mind immediately before my hospitalization and shortly after my release.

I even worked out how all of this could be accomplished after speaking to the school administrators and one of my own church elders about how to realize this ambition. What finally prevented me from pursuing this profession was the advice of virtually all of my family members and friends who begged me not to do this, and they all had different reasons.

The young East Indian man, whom I had met at the state hospital and had seemed to have such a great connection with me, managed to get in contact with me over the telephone. I am not sure how he managed to track down my grandmother's home telephone number. He said he was released from NARH, and that it would be nice to come over and visit with me. I was delighted to get a chance to talk to him and arranged for him to meet me at my apartment. When he came, I was somewhat surprised when he drove up in what appeared to be a very expensive sports car. I assumed from this that he had very supportive parents who were able to afford to provide him with this kind of vehicle.

He said that he was planning to move to New York, or someplace far away from Huntsville. This was a recurring theme in my young adult life. Hardly any of my friends wanted to remain in Huntsville for very long, since they thirsted to see other parts of the world. This meant that I would spark old friendships from time to time with people who would inevitably inform me that they had been offered a job in some other area of the country, often in Atlanta, and that they would be moving.

I had no great desire to remain in Huntsville, either, and wanted very much to be able to move to another more exotic region. One aspect, though, of having a secure living arrangement in Huntsville, was that I felt very much tied to my surroundings.

I was saddened by the fact that I would not be able to spend more time with this interesting man, and regretted that we would not be able to socialize more. That same aura of greatness we shared seemed to have vanished along with the psychotic symptoms we had experienced. We chatted briefly about one another's plans, with both of us seeming to project an air of confusion about what we would do next in our lives. He said goodbye, driving off in his sports car, leaving me feeling nostalgic about my time at NARH.

BOUNCING BACK

Living in the wild world felt more stifling in its own way than the controlled confinement of state institution walls. The all-too-brief period of time I was able to spend with my East Indian friend, combined with a terrible feeling of hopelessness about my situation, kindled something inside of me that caused me to long to be back in the state hospital. On "The Hill" I had felt like a person who was in charge of his own destiny and had been looked up to by the other patients. I had even formed a romantic relationship with someone, which was something that was missing from my short life. If my readers will recall, I had a history of wanting to be at the behavioral health section of the general hospital for a time, shortly after being diagnosed with mental illness. This thought suddenly came back to me in full force, and I began to want desperately to be back in the hospital. What I was experiencing was a form of institutionalization. While this institutionalization is a good sign of the progress in the quality of care provided to people who receive mental health care, it is immensely harmful to the client, in terms of their goal to achieve greater independence. This is much like the tendency to experiment with not taking prescribed medication according to the doctor's order. It is something of "a necessary evil" in one who discovers that he has mental illness. Both these phenomena happen to a greater or lesser degree to practically all patients diagnosed with serious mental illness.

In extreme cases, one that experiences institutionalization might actually spend his entire life inside a mental institution or some other form of restrictive environment. It could be jail, a group home, or a nursing home. This is something that is now rare because of new and improved medications, and because of a new emphasis on those with mental illness having greater freedom. This emphasis on greater freedom is affected as much by society's desire to control mental health costs as anything else. Research has shown repeatedly that it is far less expensive to provide a person supported housing in the community than it is to keep them in an institution.

It was not long ago, perhaps maybe a century ago, that one with mental illness was expected to spend his entire life inside a mental institution. These institutions were self-enclosed and self-sustaining hospital compounds, where everyone had to work in order to maintain the institution. Many people lived their entire adult lives inside the walls of these institutions, and many people died and were buried inside these enclosed cities.

Incidentally, many people who had no mental illness whatsoever also lived inside these compounds, as well. They may have had the bad luck of being arrested for an infraction considered outside the norm, and they could be committed for the rest of their lives because of that infraction. Some husbands would have their wives committed to these institutions, simply as a convenient way of depositing them in some place other than their own homes.

At that time, if one found himself in a situation like this, chances were very great that he might never escape it. Some took unneeded medications, and that may not have helped. Many experienced side effects that could be as bad, if not worse, than the real or imaginary symptoms initially experienced. The medications prescribed today have vastly improved since then.

The 1990's were called the decade of the brain because of the remarkable breakthroughs made in medications. Amazingly, scientists discovered these medications despite very small profit margins; the majority of those with serious mental illness have few resources. Additionally, government funding has been small. These medical breakthroughs, combined with improvements in client care, as well as much stricter guidelines about who could lose their freedom, progressed in fits and starts over the years. This created an entirely different situation for people with mental illness.

Though I only had rudimentary knowledge of this history at that point in my life, I knew that the hospital was a place I wanted to be. I began thinking of ways to get myself placed back there, so I started out with the obvious. I arranged a meeting with my therapist and simply told her that I felt that I should be placed back into the hospital. This went nowhere. My therapist informed me that I could not go back to the hospital simply because I wanted to do so. We worked instead on the underlying factors that led to my desire to be back within the hospital walls. Later, as I saw her on a weekly basis, I informed her that I was suicidal, thinking that would be a sure ticket to the hospital. Though I was deeply depressed during this time, partly due to my circumstances and partly due to the fact that I was suffering from post-psychotic depression, I was not completely suicidal. Since I had no firm plan to harm myself, she asked and I consented to sign a no harm contract. This is a written agreement in which I consented to do no harm to myself, and affirmed that I would contact my therapist or some other representative of the mental health center before attempting suicide. I could not fully envision actually doing physical damage to myself at that time. The no harm contract did have a kind of subconscious magic to it, which reinforced my will to live.

I stayed mostly isolated and smoked a lot of cigarettes. I felt the walls of my apartment closing in on me. I began to think that maybe I could cause some kind of public disruption, so that I would have to be confined to the hospital. The idea began turning in my mind that I should break a pane of glass in front of one of the case managers who worked at the apartment complex. I brooded for long hours on ways to do this, envisioning myself picking up the tall floor lamp I owned and dashing it into the glass of one of the apartments in the building facing the building I lived in. I stared out of the screen door of my upstairs apartment trying to will myself to commit this aggressive act. Perhaps it was the look of fear that I envisioned on the case manager's face if I carried out such a deed which finally prevented me from doing it. In any case, I could not will myself to carry out this act of sabotage, despite an enormous amount of contemplation.

I believe it was on a Sunday during this time that I came up with what I thought was an appropriate solution to my dilemma. I would simply travel to the mental health center on that day when no one was around and do some damage to it. Since I had no car, I walked on a beautiful Sunday afternoon, either from my grandmother's house, which I visited frequently, or from my apartment, to the mental health center.

Despite my recess from exercise, I did not tire during my trek. My mind firmly fixed on my plan, I finally arrived at the mental health center and walked to the outside of the Day Treatment area, which I knew well. The park benches were in front where I congregated with the other people with mental illness who attended the program.

The HMCMHC, at that time, was in a building constructed very much like a maze, with each portion looking strikingly different from the rest. The portion I now stood in front of holding a very large rock in my hand looked much like a pyramid. I once climbed to the top of this pyramid with a young man who had serious emotional problems. He ended up dying in jail at the hands of an inmate. None of this crossed my mind at this point. All I could focus on was that it would take only an instant and I would once again be free, in the inner confines of institutions.

I aimed at the large pane of glass that comprised the wall of one side of the pyramid and threw with all my strength. This was when something unexpected happened. The rock hit the pane of glass and bounced off without causing a bit of damage to it. I stood amazed as I watched the glass vibrate while the rock fell seemingly very slowly to the ground.

As one with a history of trying to watch the signs of fate, due in no small measure to my mental illness, I did not need more confirmation that I should give up this idea immediately and continue with my life as before. Whatever that glass was composed of, it was obviously made of sterner stuff than I had credited it with.

In retrospect, I realize how extremely awful any of these acts of sabotage would have been, not only to any bystanders or to the owners of the property, but to my entire future. What would likely have happened after I destroyed any of these glass windows was that I would have been arrested and sent to jail, and if lucky, would have been sent to a hospital for people with mental illness who have committed a crime. These hospitals are very highly restrictive, and similar in many respects to a prison. I have seen many other patients since that time, many of which had similar ideas, and many of which had no control of their actions, whatsoever. In their situations, whatever force that prevented me from committing an act of destruction to physical property did not prevent them from doing so. These people ended up in criminal hospitals or jails, and they did have a very difficult time regaining their freedom. I am talking here about a matter of years, at the very least.

One result of my experience with that rock is that when I meet someone with mental illness who has committed a crime and has been in an institution for the criminally "insane," I am far less likely to pass judgment on him, no matter what the crime. There is a very real aspect of my personality when dealing with them that whispers to me, "There but for the grace of God go I." Furthermore, experience has also proven that practically all people with serious mental illness seem to share this same understanding. They tend not to demonize those who commit crimes or judge them as harshly as others often do.

Another myth commonly associated with those with mental illness is that their ranks are filled with people who just managed to "plead insanity" successfully in order to beat their case. The truth is, while there are many people who try to plead insanity in criminal trials, only about one percent of the people who do plead insanity succeed in their attempt to do so. In many instances, people who succeed in pleading insanity may actually lose their freedom for a longer span of time. Fortunately for me, I was not in the ranks of those with mental illness trying to sort out their lives in the legal system. The future course of my years was altered irrevocably the instant I saw that rock bounce from the glass wall of the mental health center and fall to the ground. The people who cared for the grounds of the mental health center, who were usually young men about my age or a little younger, may have kicked that rock aside while they worked, never expecting that rock had such significance to my life.

LABOR PARTY

I'm pedaling slowly up a hill somewhere in central Louisiana. The vegetation is thick on either side of me, as is the air I'm breathing. I drank heavily the night before in a hole-in-the-wall bar in Shreveport. In Louisiana, you don't even have to be twenty-one to drink. My head now feels like it is stuffed with wet, steaming straw from the resulting hangover, and my wheels are literally moving as slow as the laws of physics will allow while still holding my frame aloft. All of a sudden, I realize that they have stopped going fast enough as I feel my body spilling off the bicycle and into the street.

"Ah, hell," I say to myself as I climb back on the bicycle and resume pedaling. At just that moment, an enormous eighteen-wheeler flies up the hill beside me. I feel the rush of air from its velocity slam into me. "Wow," I say to myself. "If that thing had been coming up the road just a few moments earlier, I'd be dead now."

One day my stepfather decided to see what my apartment was like. "This looks like a fine room," he said upon his inspection. "What would you think about me buying you a car?" he asked.

I was overjoyed, as one might imagine, considering I had not been behind the wheel for about four months. I had learned the lesson that any kind of car was a major luxury, and left the search for a car in my stepfather's hands. I was grateful when he told me that he had found a car he would like us to look at. It was a two-door Nissan and it passed his assessment. He handed the seller seven hundred dollars and the next thing I knew I was holding the title to the vehicle.

This was a tremendous gift that Dave gave me, at a time when I really needed it. Having a car was the difference between having to walk everywhere I wanted to go and enjoying the comfort of "flying down the road." The first time I drove it, after so much time away from the road, was a very strange experience.

It took a few days to get used to the hum of the machinery and to re-acquaint myself with driving. The knowledge of how difficult it would be to replace this convenience if anything happened to it shifted my compulsion to drive safely into overdrive.

I pledged to myself, and to the car, that I would drive defensively at all costs. I "rolled" to the Day Treatment program in my own car, which I decided quickly was immeasurably preferable to taking the bus.

After a few months of living in my own apartment and attending Day Treatment, I was ready to focus all of my energy on trying to make something of my future.

I had heard through my friends in the mental health community about a program called Vocational Rehabilitation Services (VRS) available to those with disabilities. The purpose was to help them find gainful employment. I heard that in many instances the program would even help pay for graduate school, if one was eligible to attend.

I quickly inquired about this program to my therapist and begged her to refer me to it. Marilyn was still relatively new to being a therapist, although she tended to move rather quickly through the ranks, since she had a wealth of business and public relations experience before she decided to devote her life to a helping profession.

When I asked her about VRS, she told me that she had not had the opportunity to learn much about the program. She did some investigating and found out that one of the people she graduated with was actually the new manager of the VRS in Huntsville. She felt very optimistic about the program and soon referred me.

I kept an appointment at a local state office where I was interviewed and filled out an application for services. I did my best to impress the woman I met there, who was an older Caucasian lady nearing retirement. Her drab dress and plain looking gray hair were worn like a badge to belie her status as a bureaucrat. She possessed an aura of business-like efficiency which in no way revealed some modicum of concern with what my experience with VRS might actually be like. She gave me surprisingly little information and avoided my questions in a practiced manner. I did learn that VRS was a state program, but that was about all the information I gleaned from the interview. She directed me to the main headquarters of VRS, located only a few blocks from where I lived.

When I went to the main headquarters, I met another woman who seemed to have a sunnier disposition who said she was in charge of testing. She gave me a battery of written and physical tests. The testing took a couple of days and I felt that the results were likely to indicate that my aptitude was about the same or higher than the average person.

Immediately following my testing, I was introduced to the man who had graduated with his Master's Degree in Counseling Psychology with Marilyn. He was a tall black man and he introduced me to another tall black man who would be my counselor in the program. This counselor had a bachelor's degree in a helping field but had not yet earned his master's.

I could readily tell that the master's level friend of my therapist was very new to his position, and was still learning the job. The other man who looked very much like Paul Harvey informed me that I was to be placed in a program in which I would do assembly work and would be observed for a time. After that, he would assist me in finding a job. This was an entirely different outcome than what I had in mind, but I agreed, reluctantly, to go along with his plan.

My steady stream of questions regarding how I would benefit from the program were still being deftly evaded, and I was receiving no answers. Although I had visions of someone helping me create my own resume or helping me enroll in graduate school, insisting these were the services that would help me, these men insisted that I participate in the manual labor program, ignoring my objections.

I had done a number of physically intensive jobs ever since I was sixteen years old. I had worked bagging groceries for my first summer job. The next summer, I cleaned rooms at a hotel managed by my sister, the summer before my first year of college. I spent the summer after my first year of college working in a factory that manufactured bathtubs and other plumbing accessories. I was no stranger to work, and knew already that I was capable of doing manual labor.

My disappointment from hearing of people who completed the program only to be referred to jobs bussing tables at the Space and Rocket Museum was palpable. I had already spent time bussing tables at a job during college for a short time. I needed no special assistance or training in acquiring a similar job. I wanted a job commensurate with my level of education, since I was a college graduate.

What I was introduced to in this program felt to me like a chamber of horrors. One of the visions I had during my first psychotic break was of being introduced to a hellish factory. My new predicament was startlingly similar to this vision, and had the effect of unnerving me considerably. The factory that I and other novices to this program worked in was on one half of the building. The other half was used by a full working factory where people operated sewing machines, making American flags.

This factory had two distinctions. The first one was that it is the only plant in America today that sews American flags. The other distinction is that it is located in the historic mill district. Most of the mills have been torn down to be replaced by green soccer fields. I often wonder how many people are aware that one sewing mill still exists there, and that many of the people who work there have mental and physical disabilities.

I was put to work boxing wires, instructional manuals, and other items for for-profit electronics companies that had contracts with VRS. I also moved pallets, taped boxes, and did any number of tasks that required little skill. I was surrounded with many people with disabilities much more severe than my own. They were pressured by the staff to finish their work quotas, as was I. These people had even less choice than I did at having to be there, since they most likely had family members who made their decisions for them.

After about a week of this labor, I was completely shocked when I saw that my first check contained alarmingly little money. I was paid a few pennies a piece for what I produced, and the number of pieces that I produced was determined by my counselor. One week's worth of labor for six hours a day resulted in a check for about twenty dollars—much less than the minimum wage of any time period I ever worked in, including the time when I helped to construct satellite dishes in the country, at age seven.

It felt to me as if I were working in a sweatshop. The thought of laboring further in these conditions was abhorrent, and I would no longer be part of it.

I told the staff at VRS and my therapist that I would not be returning to that facility, I and was surprised one day shortly thereafter when the two men I knew who operated VRS came to my apartment, sat down, and began trying to convince me that I should return to the program. They talked me into returning to the job for another three weeks. This stands high on my list of the worst experiences of my existence and I would never wish it on another living being.

Twelve years later, my outrage at what I experienced has cooled, to a certain degree. I see it as a valuable lesson as to what people are capable of doing to one another. A couple of years after this experience, I ran into the bachelor level counselor at the bank. It was the sheer force of my will that prevented me from assaulting this man physically, and I am sure he likely attributed the look of rage on my face to symptoms of my illness. I have never been, however, more in my right frame of mind, and I have never, as a rule, been prone to fits of rage. I was taken advantage of, and I resented it tremendously, as I feel most people in that position would have, as well.

After one month of laboring for almost no wages, I became so depressed about my situation that I was suicidal. I tried to hang myself with my belt, by jamming the strap into the frame of my door. I did this repeatedly, and even blacked out one time; but my fall to the floor dislodged the belt. I placed knives to my wrists and tried, but could not make myself cut very deeply. If I'd had access to firearms, such as the ones I used to own, there is very little doubt that I would be dead now.

I described my suicidal gestures to Marilyn and she referred me to the behavioral medicine wing of Huntsville Hospital once more. The female psychotherapist that assessed me for admission there said that I was acting childish and that I had no real reason to feel suicidal. She said that she had worked at McDonald's while she went through college and that I did not know how difficult life could actually be. Her initial reaction was to not admit me to the hospital, but after speaking with Marilyn, decided I should be admitted, after all.

I think that a person who assesses an individual for suicidal tendencies has a sacred trust. It is crucial for the professional in this position to try to put himself or herself in the place of the individual at risk of self-harm. The assessor should never think about what he or she would or would not do, but what the person being assessed is likely to do. The life of the individual is more important than any notion of the medical professional regarding what a person should or shouldn't be upset about. I could have made the argument to the lady assessing me that working at McDonalds was infinitely superior to working for twenty dollars per week anywhere, but the fact that I was feeling seriously suicidal would have remained in place no matter what was said by either of us. Later on in my life, I would encounter hundreds of people who told me they were feeling suicidal, and I took every one of them seriously. Their lives were too important to me to do any less.

This point in the story marks another milestone in my life. It was the last time that I was ever suicidal, as well as the last time I had to be admitted to a psychiatric hospital. It was 1999 and I had managed to survive a series of emotional challenges which could have easily cost me my life.

THE HOME FRONT

While I was a patient in the hospital, the psychiatrist there changed my medication from Risperdal to Seroquel. I still use this drug, but in the early months of 1999, I continued to hide the fact that I did not take the medicine, unless I was monitored in a structured setting.

I spent about a week in Huntsville Hospital this last time, where I wanted to spend all of my time sleeping in my room. The hospital staff did not allow this, though, and I was prodded to attend various group sessions. I was wheeled out of the hospital in a rolling chair, as that was the hospital policy at that time, even though I was perfectly capable of walking on my own. Derrick, the case manager who worked in Day Treatment, took me to a group home. A group home, I discovered, was a place where People with Mental illness who had more intensive problems, preventing them from living independently, lived for long periods. I was in what was known as the Respite program, because I was only expected to remain in the group home for a couple of weeks to a month. Derrick had a way of making connections with me and the other clients, providing encouragement and remaining professional at the same time. One thing I learned from this man during my stay at the group home was that there were instances when the staff were forced to take clients to live at the homeless shelter if they had nowhere else to go. This came up in a discussion in which I wondered what might happen if a client was behaving less than responsibly and had nowhere to stay. I was somewhat shocked to discover that if a client somehow "burned all his bridges," that the rescue mission could be a last resort.

In time, I learned that, in fact, many CMHS live in the mission by their own choice. Some CMHS feel like they have more freedom there than they do in the group homes, especially if they are unable to maintain independent living arrangements.

I was happy to have a place to stay in the group home and felt very recalcitrant about returning to my own apartment.

The group home seemed to contain an air of peaceful living that made it irresistible at that particular time in my life. I had a roommate and lived with the other people who resided at the group home and the various staff. The house where I lived was located in a cluster of about five homes located immediately behind my apartments and one of the rescue missions. On weekday mornings, the residents of the group homes would attend Day Treatment in a building that served as a community-meeting place called the Triana Life Center, after the street that intersected it. This Day Treatment program, called TLC for short, was not the same as the one I had attended previously. One memorable aspect of my attendance at TLC was a counselor on the staff named Terry, who had a mental illness of her own. She spoke openly about her own recovery.

Unlike the vast majority of the clients in this program, Terry had a severe tremor. Her head shook with every word she spoke, yet there was undeniable power in the messages she conveyed to her audience.

She gave off an aura of being much more conservative in terms of her expectations of other clients than did the other counselors I had encountered. The fact that she was in this job was testimony to the fact that PLMI were capable of obtaining their personal goals, and she had no qualms about pointing this out to people in her trembling, but penetrating, voice.

Another instance that comes to mind from the Day Treatment experience at TLC, was sitting alone on one of the picnic benches at the back of the building. I was smoking cigarettes and feeling profoundly depressed.

For some reason it really came to me, that instant, just how far I had sunk with regard to what I had planned for my life, and how the reality had taken shape. The surrealism of my situation hit me like a shovel, and in many ways I felt like this must have been the lowest point of my life. There was very little room for hope in my mindset at that time, and thoughts of what I would do once I moved out of the group home were pushed further into the background of my mind.

In the last two and a half years since my first psychotic break, a time that had been punctuated with numbing despair as well as mind shattering experiences, this moment of relative comfort and safety felt like one of the lowest points of all.

This feeling of supreme desolation made me even more grateful that I had a place like the Respite program, where I could get away from it all. I took so readily to the group home life that there was a very big part of me that did not want to ever move back to my apartment. I discovered that I was not alone in feeling this way. Most of the people living with me were very content to be there, and almost none of them seemed in any particular hurry to get out. It was a very relaxing environment, and after what I had experienced prior to my hospitalization, the slow but steady pace of the group home really appealed to me.

We ate breakfast, lunch, and dinner at the same time every day, and I considered the food well prepared. We had to do light chores around the home. After Day Treatment, we socialized. We smoked one cigarette every hour under supervision, and watched television.

The woman who managed the group home really cared about all of the residents. She was not able to be around the home all the time however, since she undoubtedly had other homes she had to administer. She was black, like most of the women who worked at the home. And she seemed to have a charisma that transcended race and gender when she worked with the residents.

One day, she told me that there was an Annual Consumer Conference held in Talladega, Alabama that I might be interested in attending. She did not provide many details about what the conference was, exactly, other than the date of the event, which was two months away. She convinced me to sign up and pay my ten-dollar fee for attendance, and repeated her assurances that I would enjoy the conference.

A great source of inspiration and recreation for all residents was a spiritual meeting we attended about once every two weeks. Food and prayer were shared by all, as people with mental illness from across the community attended the function and enjoyed fellowship with one another. These meetings took place in a section of the Vocational Rehabilitation Services building that had been the source of so much difficulty for me. As I tried to put the bad memories aside, it was certainly good to be in that building for a purpose other than for the reason I had been there initially.

After about six weeks of living in the group home, I was gently nudged by the charismatic group home manager back to my apartment for one day, in an attempt to recondition myself to living there. She told me I was ready to be back in my own apartment. I walked back to my apartment and opened the door and there were fourteen messages on my telephone. I listened to these feeling overwhelmed by the effort of processing them. I managed to stay there for one night, and I was grateful to return to the group home for one more day. After that day I returned to my own place feeling moderately prepared to try and figure out what to do with the rest of my life.

The time spent in the group home had been beneficial, and after a couple of days back in my own place, I felt good about living there again. The desire I'd had to be institutionalized in a restrictive environment was banished. I made up my mind to make my way in life as independently as I could. I was not in law school as I'd planned, but at least I had privacy while I attempted to fit the pieces of my broken life into some sort of discernable pattern. While this was a long endeavor, fraught with all manner of unforeseen pitfalls, I was aided in my efforts by the fact that I never again required the intense structure inherent in life at places like the hospital and group home.

HOME AWAY FROM HOME

Once again, I was traveling to the HMCMHC in my car to attend the Day Treatment program there. One surprising development that occurred during this time was my appointment to the Consumer Council at the HMCMHC.

The reason why this appointment was surprising was that I was the youngest member on the Consumer Council. The other members of the council had been there for some time, and they wore the hardships of surviving with serious mental illness, decade after decade, on their faces like finely polished masks.

Some of the six members, other than me, lived on their own while others lived in permanent group homes. The primary purpose of the Consumer Council was to give the clients of the HMCMHC a voice in the operations of the organization.

Meetings were once a month and gave me further opportunity to interact with people who had successfully coped with the best and worst that the mental health system in Alabama had to offer through the years. The main discussion of the council, at that point, focused on providing support for one another. It was an honorary position and no serious discussion on mental health center policy was ever had. I could not figure out why I was chosen to have a place with people who had endured so much, while I was decades younger and still struggling with my own identity.

One member of the Consumer Council was a man in his late fifties, named Louis Brackeen. He had been the president of the Manic Depressive Support Group for some time. Before the onset of his illness, he was a married executive of a bank in Auburn, Alabama. Now he was a single man who focused all of his energy on maintaining his recovery from his illness, and supporting other people in their efforts to do so. He was kind enough to provide me transportation to the Consumer Conference in Talladega. I accepted his offer and we drove through miles of open country in order to reach the Shocco Springs Baptist Conference Center.

I had no real idea about what the Consumer Conference was about. All I knew about it was that it was something related to mental health. I knew this because the manager of the group home I had lived in had encouraged me to fill out the application form for the conference a couple of months earlier.

Located in an Eden of natural splendor, Shocco Springs was the site of many religious retreats. The large central building, which served as the compound's nerve center, contained ping pong tables, conference rooms, and galleries displaying works of art created by PLMI.

A Christian gift shop and bookstore attached to this building had a steady flow of customers. Another point of interest in this building was the gigantic cafeteria, which had a seemingly-inexhaustible capability to seat and feed hundreds of people. The quality of food was superb. This central building connected to a number of buildings on both sides that formed a sort of semi-circle. These vast buildings all contained several floors that were virtually hotel rooms. But they were somewhat different from typical hotel rooms in that they contained no televisions, no telephones, and no amenities, such as soap or shampoo.

The first thing I encountered as Louis and I arrived was about one hundred people congregating around tables filled with sugar cookies and lemonade. Louis introduced me to a number of people he knew, and in short order I found myself feeling at home in my surroundings. I soon began to explore the area on my own and discovered that there were PLMI of all ages, and on all levels of functioning.

People from mental health centers from all across Alabama and other states had come to the Consumer Conference. It was not long before we went into a chapel area where the opening sessions were held. Ashtrays, which usually were not necessary, were placed everywhere in an attempt to preserve the neat appearance of the grounds, because the majority of the attendees smoked.

The opening ceremonies were of a spiritual nature, and I was surprised to find that the Serenity Prayer was a part of the services. The

Serenity Prayer is usually associated with Alcoholics Anonymous. For anyone who is not familiar with it, the prayer goes like this. "God grant me the serenity to accept the things I cannot change, the courage to change the things I can, and the wisdom to know the difference."

The white-haired spiritual leader of the Conference, conducting this phase of the gathering, seemed to believe that the Serenity Prayer was an equally powerful instrument for addressing the needs of PLMI, who were not necessarily associated with Alcoholics Anonymous.

I won't attempt describe all aspects of the conference, for there is no substitute for actual attendance. There were amazing educators and speakers, speaking on a wide array of issues that affect PLMI. Additionally, participants had the opportunity to socialize and spend time with one another, learning from each other's experiences ways to be successful in recovery.

But I came to understand that the most powerful and important component of the movement is spirituality. It was the force meshing the tiny individual voices of PLMI into one powerful whole.

At the conference, a man came to speak who declared that a new day had dawned for those who receive mental health services in Alabama, and, throughout the country.

He was the attorney, James Tucker, and he represented the Alabama Disabilities Advocacy Program (ADAP). The new day he spoke of was because of a landmark legal case, supported by ADAP, that brought powerful changes to the lives of people throughout the state and country. Tucker explained that this epic case was settled after decades of court battles in succeeding waves over the decades, ushering in new and larger reforms with each phase of its resolution.

I began to understand, then, that this was the reason why my treatment at the state hospital had been so pleasant, instead of the nightmarish visions some see when thinking about mental institutions. These laws were the reason I was allowed to have an apartment as well as other resources available for my treatment.

In fact, the changes were the reason I was able to stand at this conference I was attending for PLMI, and hear the remarkable words from the man I was listening to.

The name of this legal case was Wyatt vs. Stickney, and it was the first of its kind. One can find the details of Wyatt vs. Stickney in any modern textbook related to social welfare and mental health issues. It transformed the state of Alabama into a model state in terms of mental health care, which other states are now trying to copy.

Fifteen-year-old Ricky Wyatt suffered the abuses of an inhumane system in Bryce Hospital and filed suit against the state in 1970. ADAP represented Ricky Wyatt and the thousands of other PLMI in the state of Alabama he symbolized. The outcome of the lawsuit created sweeping changes to provide for the treatment and social welfare for PLMI in Alabama.

My astonishment and happiness were tempered by a sense of sadness as I realized that my mother did not live to see these reforms that could have improved her life. She died at thirty-nine without a fraction of the benefits I now had, from modern medication to the rights to raise her own children in a stable environment.

As I sat in that crowd listening to James Tucker's words, I realized again that many of the people filling those seats had lived through the same deprivations as my mother, but they had managed, by some great miracle, to survive. When one lives in the dawning of a new age they rub elbows with some highly esteemed company.

I rode home with Louis, grateful for the experience of attending the annual Consumer Conference at Shocco Springs.

Life at my apartment now found me spending time with others who I would not likely have had the opportunity to meet, had I not experienced having mental illness. One in particular was a down-on-his-luck black man in his middle age named Ezel, who I have described in some detail, previously.

I do not know why I enjoyed spending the amount of time with Ezel that I did, however I found myself at his apartment quite frequently. We would attend Day Treatment at the mental health center during the day, two or three times a week, and we had really very little else to do to fill the rest of our hours.

I would walk across the apartment complex to his place in the afternoons and watch television. He really did not care much about what we watched, and often he would cook chicken wings or some other tasty confection. He was very proud of showing off his cooking degrees. He had earned these earlier in his life, when times were better, and now had them locked away in a metal box.

Ezel tended to drink a great deal more than I did, and had some ability to become a completely different, and far less likeable, person whenever he did so. I once took him to the bar I enjoyed "hanging out" in. He enjoyed the good music, and I enjoyed watching him "cut a rug" with the best of them.

The time I spent with Ezel began to dwindle as I began spending time on other pursuits, described later. At some point down the line, Ezel took a turn for the worse and began spending time with a seedier group of people. I will never forget awaking one morning to see his entire apartment building engulfed in flames, and the unfortunate residents it housed milling around the blaze. The Huntsville News, decided to quote me when I told them that "it looked like a giant bonfire."

Ezel disappeared from Shelter Plus after that, but eventually moved into another apartment. I had the chance to visit him on a couple of occasions. When I last saw him, he had completely reformed his ways of living and had returned to work, and even remarried. I never will forget Ezel, and I hope very much to see him again one of these days.

I kept a watch on my grandmother. Bert still lived with her and provided her care. One time, I remember going there and saw my brother and a number of his friends sitting around and joking. This was a surreal experience for me, I'd had my home at my grandmother's side for so long. I had recurring nightmares about him displacing me from my home for years after it actually happened.

In my regular conversations with my grandmother, I discovered that things were not working out with Bert living there. He was demonstrating more and more symptoms related to his mental illness and was finding it increasingly difficult to mask these from my grandmother.

I knew enough about mental health to try to explain to her what was going on with Bert, but she ignored my explanations. She was in a state of denial about what Bert was experiencing. She said he had gone to our family doctor who had examined him and prescribed him what he needed. The doctor gave him a prescription for Ativan, a mild sleeping drug. I tried to explain to her that he needed something much more potent, like an antipsychotic medication. My advice was ignored, and Bert's symptoms became more pronounced. This was very frustrating to me because I felt like I was trying to argue something obvious to someone who simply didn't want to believe what I had to say.

My grandmother, now in her mid-eighties, was becoming incapable of understanding the reality of the situation. Disaster seemed immanent to me, but there was really nothing I could do except watch and be ready for whenever the house of cards began its inevitable fall. I also considered myself extraordinarily lucky that I no longer had to live in that environment.

I had recognized the impracticality of my grandmother and brother's living arrangement from the beginning. How, after all, could they expect my stepfather to keep providing their living expenses in a house that he paid the mortgage on, for any length of time. This situation became worse when my grandmother told me that my stepfather was going to have heart surgery. Now, as he prepared for the operation, he would be even less capable of addressing the situation than he had been before I had moved out of the house.

I visited him occasionally at his house. He explained, in detail, the surgery he was having, and we would discuss the nature of life in general. My views tended to lean a bit more toward religion than his did. I enjoyed these visits with him and did everything I could to encourage him in the days leading up to his operation.

SAFETIES AND SECURITIES

I discovered by mail that I would no longer receive disability payments, though the letter did not say why. After speaking with my therapist, Marilyn, about this, I discovered it was because my case manager did not fill out some form that she was supposed to send back to the Social Security Administration. This, incidentally, was the same case manager I had contemplated scaring in order to be readmitted to the hospital.

Marilyn highly recommended that I reapply immediately in order to resume disability payments. All I could envision was the immediate resulting lack of money I was used to collecting each month, and I dreaded slipping further into poverty. Perhaps, I thought, my grandmother had been correct all along, and there was no way the government was going to provide adequate money for my living expenses.

"I have to find a job," I said to myself.

I began looking through the newspaper for job listings. I knew for certain that I did not prefer working at a manual labor job. At one point during my search, I applied at the state hospital where I had resided. I was required to take a state test in order to do so, and thought I did quite well. However, I never received a call for an interview. I applied to many other places, as well, but the job that I managed to find right away was in security.

My first posting as a security officer was for a place that contracted services for the General Electric plant in Decatur. It was a long drive, although I enjoyed the rather leisurely pace afforded by the position. I would spend some hours sitting in the small hut outside the plant, waiting to log eighteen-wheeler trucks and other vehicles in and out of the facility. At other times, I walked on what were called "key rounds."

In these, I drove a golf cart around the plant and placed a handheld device that electronically registered my visit. I was mystified to see the mysterious machinery and inner workings of the plant.

One aspect of working as a security guard was that I constantly had to work different shifts. Working on the third shift, which was from midnight until morning, was interesting, since there was little activity going on in the plant during those hours. It was refreshing to be able to sit down read a book and get paid, though poorly, to do the job.

It also felt good to be back in the town in which I was institutionalized, but for an entirely different reason. On a few occasions, I was sent to the new Boeing rocket plant being built in Decatur. Things were very quiet there, and I didn't have to leave the hut at all. Boeing did not even want the security officers to trespass on their property.

I was not working in security long before I encountered one of my friends who lived in the same housing program as me. She asked if I wanted a job doing security work at the local mall, since I was already in that line of work. I jumped at this opportunity, and after two weeks of doing security work, I found a job paying seven dollars an hour at a place only a few miles away from my home, in contrast to making minimum wage in a different city.

Though the River City of Decatur is much smaller than the Rocket City of Huntsville now, it was actually larger than Huntsville until the early nineteen sixties.

My grandmother was a very prominent woman in the Huntsville community in the sixties and seventies, as the Secretary of the Expansion Committee of the Huntsville Chamber of Commerce. For twelve years, she worked diligently helping to make Huntsville a growing city, working along with partners to attract the National Aeronautics and Space Administration (NASA). The space shuttle and many of NASA's rockets are designed and built in Huntsville. This led to Huntsville evolving into the Silicon Valley of the South. This work had a rippling effect on Decatur, which hosts Boeing and other aerospace companies.

My grandmother's appointment to this position of responsibility was one afforded to relatively few women in her generation. Although she was transformed by time and tragedy by the time she made the decision to take on the task of raising me, the iron underneath the surface of her persona never really faded. It seems now that her decision late in life to raise a child, who had clearly suffered emotionally from his initial childhood experiences, was one more of her extraordinary accomplishments.

One effect my upbringing has had on me is that I admire and respect women in positions of authority. In my experience, many men can seem annoyed at having women command them.

Whenever I feel tempted to feel that way myself, I do not have to think very deeply to remember my grandmother, and the strength that she held in her position of authority. She had the extraordinary ability to bolster her community and make sure all feel welcome, while at the same time, she did everything she could to ensure the security and continuity of her own family.

She remains one of the two most saintly people I have ever met. My stepfather is the other person with a similar character. This quality, as much as anything, kept the tattered fragments of my family together, for as long as it was.

She spent her entire fortune in trying to keep my mother alive and healthy. She spent vast sums of money on psychiatric hospitals and doctor's bills for my mother's care. In the nineteen seventies, insurance companies did not provide health care coverage for mental health care to the same extent as physical health care. This problem is still being hotly debated to this day, as people have to file bankruptcy due to gigantic hospital bills. In 1974, when my grandmother began to feel hard hit financially, this debate was nowhere close to the forefront of public consciousness.

By the time I came into my grandmother's life, the majority of her economic resources had been spent on her attempt to save my mother's life. Her love and grace then were my sustenance, as much as anything else we shared together in our relationship with one another.

My stepfather's infinite capacity for compassion and reason sustained me, as did his financial backing. He always seemed to place everything else ahead of his own material wants.

This duo maintained their place as the titans of my upbringing and development. I think they were surprised to see me working as a security officer after graduating from college and I know it was a line of work that I did not expect to be in.

At the Parkway City Mall, I learned an entirely different form of security work. I discovered that the difference in the security work I did at the mall and the type of security work I did at the General Electric plant was primarily a matter of public relations.

At the General Electric plant, the majority of the work that I did was in the shadows, outside the public eye, inside the inner recesses of the plant where very few people traveled, and none of them were interested in spending time with me.

It was almost eerie that I could stand in the same break room as the people who worked in the plant, yet if I came upon one or a pair of them there, it was as if I were merely a phantom lurking just beyond awareness. At the mall, though, I was not only expected to be in the public eye, but I also constantly had to deal with many types of people. I had to wear a very eye-catching uniform, which included a large wide brimmed hat.

To be in the public eye was a double-edged sword. I had the opportunity to engage socially with many people, but I was very self-conscious about being a security officer, especially in a situation that was so conspicuous.

The high school that I graduated from was located practically right next door to the mall, and most of the people I graduated with had gone on to work at high-paying jobs. Whenever I ran into someone I knew, a streak of shame would instantly rise in me because I worked at a menial job.

I felt there was another me out there, who never had a mental illness, living some other existence. In that man's reality, working as a security officer at the mall was simply not an option.

This line of thinking struck me primarily in the morning when I had to open the doors to the mall for the walking crowd, who were mostly elderly people.

I said to myself, "These people must really look down on me for having to work as the mall security guard."

In retrospect, I realize that this way of thinking was based, for the most part, on my youth. The truth was that working at this job was good for my personal growth. I provided genuine help to people from time to time, and I had the opportunity to meet and socialize with people, despite the chagrin related to my role. Having to follow work rules and focus on specific tasks helped to forge a sense of self-discipline in me.

Since I had lost my disability payments, I did not have to pay rent for my apartment, which had been thirty percent of my income. I was not asked, initially, to resume my rent payments after getting my job. The net result was that I had quite a bit more income than I had previously when I received a disability check.

I was working at this job for about eight months when I met a woman, whom I will call Jane Anne, and began dating her. It felt very good and somewhat surreal to be with her after being in romantic limbo for such a long time. I did not foresee a long-term relationship with her, though, and was in a constant tug of war with her about this from the beginning.

When I discussed this situation with my therapist, Marilyn, I expected her to understand my feelings about this and immediately take my side. I was wrong. I immediately found that my therapist's view was in startling contrast to what my fraternity brothers' opinions would have been.

"You shouldn't be kissing on someone you are not serious about," she said.

I have always been a person of conscience, or what therapists would term, a person with a large superego. This virtue had not penetrated my thoughts as they related to dating, mainly because I did not have opportunity to date as much as I would have liked. The men I knew never seemed to consider the feelings of the women they dated.

While I did not immediately end my relationship with Jane Anne, my therapist's words gave me more insight and empathy in my choices in relationships.

I stopped speaking to Jane Anne after about six weeks, thinking that the relationship had really reached a dead end.

One byproduct of working as a security officer was that I managed to renew my efforts at maintaining my weight. Constantly walking around the mall increased my level of physical fitness tremendously, and I watched my waistline shrink once again. I experimented with different diets in an effort to augment my physical exercise.

Aside from my feelings of awkwardness from what I considered a diminished social status, events really began going more in my favor. If my return to the workforce found me on what I considered to be at the bottom of the totem pole, at least it allowed me to once again be a part of a community that was separate from the insulated mental health world.

Once I realized that I was capable of handling the world of work, I began to dream of ways to broaden my horizons even further.

DRAINING THE SWAMP

There was no real sense of orderliness to my jumbled attempts to set my life more in line with my vision of the future, yet there was rich vitality, innocence, and a naïveté to just how brutal and nasty life can really become.

In some sense, I really didn't understand how young I was, and I put a lot of pressure on myself to succeed, and to do it quickly. These efforts lacked good direction and were often undercut by their own vitality. These attempts to break free of my circumstances comprise the rich soil that filled my life in these years. This swamp of my life would have to be drained before I could transform it into the fertile garden it would become. And it was drained by a series of family problems, to which I diverted my energy in order to solve.

It took time and patience for the man I was then to navigate the waters of tragic circumstances that strike all families and people, at one time or another. Every one of these tragedies and attempts to improve my standard of living are filled with equal parts hope and sorrow, but they all shaped me into the man I became.

My therapist, Marilyn, suggested that I may want to consider becoming a teacher, and I thought, "Why not consider that as an option?" In many ways, I felt tied to the area where I lived because of family obligations and because of my housing arrangements. I decided to visit the University of Alabama in Huntsville (UAH) to see what it could offer in the field of education.

I met with a counselor in the English Department. The white-haired male professor I met quickly dissuaded me from the idea of becoming a teacher and instead asked me to consider entering a master's program for those who wanted to become technical writers.

Companies hired technical writers to help write product manuals or other necessary documents. The Technical Writing program was a branch of the English Department, and was highly related to writing composition.

Writing composition is the study of how to write, as opposed to English Literature, which is so widely studied in English departments. The idea appealed to me immediately, and I quickly registered for the program without fully understanding what the discipline entailed. I took out a loan for my tuition and books and proudly informed my family, friends, and therapist of what I intended to do. I resigned my position at the mall so I could focus all of my attention on my studies. I felt enormously relieved to be able to lay down the ten-gallon hat, which was part of the security guard uniform. To me, it symbolized my inability to make it in the professional world. I remember purchasing my books and reveling in the syllabus, which I felt was my key to a brighter future.

One of the most dynamic changes that occurred in my life was that I had officially entered the computer age. My technical writing advisor, whom I will call Dr. Williams, told me that I had to purchase a computer and enroll in Computer Science 101.

I had already taken, and passed, Computer Science 101 seven years earlier when I was a freshman at UA. The difference, though, was that when I had taken Computer Science before, the entire subject seemed a great deal more incomprehensible than it did in 1999. A more accurate way to describe the situation was that it was now a completely different science altogether.

In 1992, understanding computers meant knowing how to write in the seemingly incomprehensible computer code necessary to execute any function. I squeaked through the class with a C primarily by understanding everything I could about the nature of the computer hardware, which was where a little less than half the points for the class were derived.

I also did much begging and pleading with other students to help me along with the labs involving the unfathomable computer code. By the end of the class, I felt so relieved at having gotten through it that I never contemplated taking another computer course until this point.

In 1999, everything was different. With the advent of Microsoft Windows, icons had replaced the ghastly computer code, and navigating the computer was less complex for the user than it had ever been before.

It was comparable to taking a class on sewing fifty years before the invention of the sewing machine, and then taking the same class five years after it had been developed. Another apt analogy would be taking a class on journalism the year before removing typewriters from the classroom and bringing in word processors—this actually occurred to me when I was a sophomore in college.

The Internet was also in common use in 1999, as it was not in 1992. I managed to cross the digital divide, which was now more traversable than ever before. At one moment I was disconnected from the world, and in the next I was completely integrated into an immeasurable volume of data and communication.

Learning to navigate the web, though, was only part of what I learned at UAH. I was there, after all, to learn more about writing, a craft I had honed in some measure during my earlier college years.

Writing about the process of writing, I learned, can be a very arduous practice. I had to find a topic related to writing that I could make my own for research.

One topic of interest to me was a field known as cognitive recording. This was, in effect, the study of measuring people's cognitions or thought patterns by utilizing various testing techniques on paper. If this topic of research sounds vague and likely difficult to find much material on, this was in fact the case, or at least it was in 1999.

The other students, who were mostly women, seemed to have little difficulty in finding topics they wanted to research and had a great deal of material supporting them. In fact, many already had technical jobs, which they could draw on for information in order to support their research.

I began to feel like I had to find some kind of employment while in school to provide additional income. I asked my technical writing advisor, Dr. Williams, if she could help me. I hoped to make an entrance into the professional work force before I completed graduate school. While her initial reaction seemed to indicate that she could not understand why I would want to work while doing intense research, she decided to help me. Her first attempt was to set up an interview at the school library for me to work as an assistant librarian. After the interview, I was informed politely that I would not be getting the job.

The next prospect Dr. Williams offered me was a non-paid internship for a firm who was designing a new software package. I was interested, because I thought that this might lead to paid employment, so I interviewed with the firm. They were more than happy to accept my services. As it turned out, they were located in a small storefront, and were working on a program to create software for medical billing. I became interested in the entire process.

I soon discovered that the firm I was with wanted me to provide an enormous amount of unpaid and tedious labor. They wanted me to create time-consuming lists of medical information and to write various pieces of literature for the company, including its mission statement.

In the meantime, I was expected to do the research required for writing several fifteen to twenty-page papers. I had difficulty wrapping my mind around cognitive recording, the complicated field of study I had elected to write the papers on, and I could only find one or two papers related to that field of study. I found myself further and further behind in gathering and processing the information I would need in order to write these lengthy papers.

Feeling overwhelmed, I made the rather unwise decision of dropping out of school altogether, without even informing my advisor. I then had to explain this decision to both my family and to my therapist. I could read in their facial expressions feelings of disappointment.

Some months later, I walked into the Huntsville Public Library just as Dr. Williams was walking out. She turned her head away from me and did not speak. I was quite embarrassed by this encounter, but was not completely shocked by her reaction.

As it turned out, though, I had other problems. These were closer to the "school of hard knocks" so frequently mentioned by people who have lived long enough to face difficult circumstances.

During the fall of 1999, I was spending a great deal of time driving back and forth from Birmingham visiting with Rob, one of my high school friends.

We spent time together on again and off again throughout our young years. Rob worked as a civil engineer for an oil pipe company, while his roommate, Jimmy, another high school friend, worked as a junior executive in an insurance firm. Their success appeared so natural, much like my friend Tommy's, that it made the tragedy of my own circumstances and the difficulty I was experiencing in obtaining a profession seem all the more palpable.

We toured Birmingham's available nightlife on occasion, and watched a lot of football together. They had graduated from Auburn and I from Alabama, but we were able to live with this difference well enough to be able to enjoy the games of both teams while together. I pursued women during these visits. I was fond of one woman in particular who lived in Birmingham, whom I will call Karen. Karen was my age and had attended the same high school. She had been successfully maintaining a career in pharmaceutical sales.

Our relationship evolved into little more than a friendship, though, it was clear to everyone that I wanted more. We met once or twice in Huntsville and Birmingham, though nothing non-platonic ever materialized. Once, we met at the movie theater in Huntsville, where we watched the new James Bond film, which was her favorite type of movie.

There was also the rather awkward date we had, in which I drove to the top of the hill, where many wealthy families lived, and became lost in the maze of expensive houses in search of her family's mansion. I finally had to stop at the family home of one of my friends from Birmingham to ask for directions.

The fact that my old friend knew I had a mental illness, and additionally, that I had not visited for years, made for a rather uncomfortable set of circumstances. After a while, I got the directions I needed to find my way to my date. Finally, late, I arrived at my date's parents' palatial home.

My heightened feelings of nervousness only became more pronounced as I met Karen's parents for the first time. I felt a wave of disapproval wash over me as I met them. The fumbling words I used to describe my family's heritage to her father, who was a doctor, sounded clownish to my own ears. I was always aware that I had no profession, and no idea of what I was going to do with my life. Neither Karen, nor her parents, knew that I had mental illness.

This was another harsh reality I had to face. Before the onset of my mental illness, parents of women I dated had always approved of me, even if I had a difficult time impressing their daughters enough to get to that point in the first place. Now that advantage was gone, at least in the case of these parents, and I was left floundering in their presence.

Karen and I spent a long time talking on the telephone, and our two groups of friends ended up spending a lot more time with one another. I had a number of other friends from Huntsville who were living in Birmingham, and I enjoyed spending time with them all. After dropping out of technical writing school, I began searching for a job, so I could fully participate in the social sphere to which I was aspiring. I planned to do this by entering the job placement program at the UA since I had graduated from the school three years before.

I thought that this was something I should have done when I first graduated from UA. The people at the program helped me to put together a resume and I used my newly acquired computer skills to apply for a number of jobs through the program.

I received interviews for a number of business jobs with corporations, including a well-known toy company, a food distribution company, and a popular sports apparel store. The interviewers were uninterested when they learned that I had not majored in a business field.

The men who interviewed me for a position as a manager in a sports apparel store, however, seemed enthusiastic about hiring me, despite my lack of formal education in business. This duo, consisting of one man in his forties and one new hire as green as me, seemed very charming and eager to have me on board their ship, up until the point when they asked about my credit history.

My credit rating was poor. I had incurred a heavy burden of hospital bills, and had been in a position where I had little or no money to pay some credit card debts I had incurred. The older leader of the two men who had been eager to hire me only a moment before, now informed me that he believed that having bad credit was evidence of a serious character flaw and dismissively terminated the interview. It became clear to me that my inability to pay the enormous medical bills I had incurred had effectively barred me from the business professions.

Feeling disillusioned, I went back to the mall "dragging my tail between my legs" and asked to get back into my old security job. My boss, Rick, was a retired military policeman from the Army. He had worked at the mall for many years. He told me that he would hire me again, but that he could not hire me back a second time if I decided to resign again.

This seemed to be some kind of universal workplace norm, and I took his words seriously. I circled the mall relentlessly, feeling embarrassed all over again for finding myself in these circumstances, yet at the same time feeling grateful for the income and physical exercise my job provided me.

My working hours ended the frequent visits to my friends in Birmingham, since I was on the clock at the mall every weekend. I maintained my relationship with them primarily over the telephone. I also maintained telephonic contact with Karen.

My grandmother told me that the date of my stepfather's long awaited heart surgery had arrived. She made it clear that Bert and I were expected to go visit my stepfather after his surgery. We marched, like two tin soldiers programmed with a sense of obligation, to the hospital to visit him as instructed.

The first person we saw upon arriving at the hospital was my stepbrother, Wendell, who was a practicing bankruptcy attorney living in Saint Louis. He appeared distraught, and his gaze seemed to penetrate us with his concern for his dad. I looked down, since my own feelings of failure at my inability to contribute to the family bubbled to the surface.

We rode that inevitable and overly large elevator up to the floor that housed the man who had been a part of our lives, in one way or another, for as long as I could remember. What I saw when I exited the elevator door was entirely unexpected. I saw my stepfather struggling to walk behind an I.V. holder he was using for support. He looked as if he had aged ten years within the course of the couple of months that it had been since I had seen him.

I hardly recognized him. Bert, appearing gaunt and ragged, as he had for some years, walked beside me as we entered my stepfather's small hospital room where Wendell escorted him to his bed. My brother and I entered the room, and somehow the role as spokesperson for my side of the family seemed to magically fall upon me. It was with this sense of profound ambassadorship that I uttered the only words that I could feel forming on my mouth.

"I'm certainly glad to see you made it through!" I said. These words sounded rather awkward to my own ears, but my ears were not so stopped up with embarrassment that I did not hear the words that he then spoke, in his sarcastic way.

"I can promise you that you are certainly no happier than I am," he said.

I then looked with something akin to astonishment into my stepbrother's eyes. He seemed to be smiling at my reaction. Even in the midst of this terrible ordeal he was undergoing, Dave managed to have the wit to teach us all something at that time. He managed to convey to all of us of what it feels like to face matters of life and death on a personal level.

My stepfather took time off from work to recuperate from his surgery and seemed to regain his vigor rapidly, although he maintained his aged appearance, for the most part. This man had been hale and hardy, even in his early sixties, never even considered smoking a cigarette, and maintained the simplest of diets.

We had all been surprised that it was necessary for him to have heart surgery, even though he was then a man in his mid-seventies. He returned to his job at the Redstone Arsenal as soon as possible.

Before his surgery, while visiting him at his house, which was part museum, part workshop, I asked him, "Why don't you simply retire?" He could have retired at any time, after working there for over thirty years.

He said, "If I retire, it will cost me about four thousand dollars a year."

I'm sure my eyes must have registered astonishment, as they usually did on hearing such answers. My stepfather earned over sixty thousand dollars a year for just about for as long as I could remember, and his personal living expenses were amazingly low. When he had found out he would have to begin paying more for cable television, he chose to live without it for years until it reached a price he was willing to pay. I was now astounded even further to hear that he would let the matter of four thousand dollars prevent him from retiring.

He had stated, many times, that he had lived through the Great Depression of the nineteen thirties, and it had altered his life irrevocably. At one point after his surgery, he was helping me with a minor car repair. He told me of a story of when he was driving his car across a bridge on bald tires and was extremely nervous that he would not make it across the bridge without getting a flat.

"Why didn't you just use the spare tire in the trunk?" I asked.

Raising the eyebrows on his face which looked very much like Albert Einstein's, he said, "Because I couldn't afford to buy a spare tire."

Although Dave was as much a self-made man as any one of us truly can be, his experiences did not make him so hard-shelled that he ever stopped considering the plight of others. Instead, they made him more attuned to the struggles of those who had lesser means. The society of conspicuous consumption that had thrived throughout my life was incomprehensible to him. He preferred to live a life of simplicity in which he consumed as few resources as he reasonably could. Thanks to his successful heart surgery, he would continue to provide valuable insight to his family for some time to come.

BRAIN DRAIN

In the winter of 2000, I still worked as a security officer at the mall. I received a phone call from Jane Anne, the woman I'd had a brief relationship with when I worked at the mall the first time. She wanted to meet with me, and I felt unable to deny her request, especially because my relationship with Karen seemed to be going nowhere fast. Jane Ann had moved to New Jersey briefly and been in a relationship with another man there. It did not work out, and she was upset with me for ending our communication as abruptly as I had. She said she was the type of person who went after what she wanted and that she wanted our relationship to be renewed.

Our relationship then began to evolve into something I considered far more serious than what it was before, and she said it had, in fact, been serious the whole time. There were worse fates in my mind, and I began growing more resigned to my role as being involved in a serious relationship with her. I had never been in a serious relationship before, although I was twenty-five years old and frankly felt I had nothing to lose in trying my hand at it. She helped rekindle my thoughts about becoming a teacher, since her parents were both in that profession, and she was studying to enter the field herself. They all convinced me that it was a profession I should consider pursuing.

Jane Anne met my grandmother and became instantly attached to her. My grandmother had a kind of magical effect on people. It was like some strange gift which allowed her access to the ears of more well-off parents. This gift of hers became more powerful and more subtle with age, and allowed me to share my childhood with their children. My girlfriend quickly began pampering and taking care of my grandmother, also a gift that I am ashamed to say that I lacked.

In the spring of 2000, after a couple of months of renewing our relationship, Jane Anne discovered one of the bottles of my antipsychotic medication that I wasn't taking in my bathroom cabinet and asked me what it was for. I then informed her that I had schizophrenia. We had known each other for about six months at that point.

A strong sense of self-preservation had guided me in my decision not to tell her anything until I had to. She was reasonably accepting, though the shock in her eyes on my admission is indelibly burned into my mind, just as it will be whenever I inform anyone of this fact again. She and her family were very understanding of my situation, though, and remained committed to the idea of me becoming a teacher. I began leaping over all the hurdles necessary to obtain a teaching career. I worked as a substitute teacher, and I consulted with advisors about obtaining the necessary education requirements.

This new responsibility led me to make a fateful life decision. I began, for a time, taking my medication on my own, without having to be hospitalized first. I made this decision when I learned that I would be responsible for dispensing medications to many of the children I would be working with. Before I took the responsibility for overseeing the care of other people, the decision to take medication was still a question open to debate, in my mind. On the one hand, I knew that I had a mental illness, and that medication could help people with this problem. On the other hand, I was not currently experiencing any symptoms, and I thought I could just begin taking medication if I did.

I was, however, not willing to gamble with the lives of other people's children by not doing everything in my power do what was expected of me. My girlfriend did not have to nudge me very far in this direction for me to see this necessity. One thing I found in my experiment of taking my medication as I was expected to was that the medication I was prescribed, Seroquel, had the side effect of making me extremely drowsy and putting me to sleep. I did not, however, experience any of the other secondary reactions that I had experienced as a twenty-one-year-old taking medication for the first time.

It was highly rewarding to teach the children as a substitute teacher in a variety of settings. I changed my mind frequently about the subjects I wanted to teach full-time, since I did everything from monitoring young children with behavioral problems to teaching language studies to middle school children. I got along well with the principals and other faculty and it seemed, for a time, that I had finally found my niche.

I wondered to myself, "Is a PLMI, who has been committed to a state hospital, even allowed to teach, or be a member of other helping professions?" After calling the Alabama State Board of Education, I discovered the answer to this question is a resounding yes! The fact that I had a disability did not bar me from entering the helping professions. If I had been convicted of a crime or had my name placed on the state sex crime registry, then I could be disqualified from employment. One who enters virtually all helping professions goes through a thorough investigation from the Federal Bureau of Investigation and state investigation agency to ensure he has not been convicted of committing an act making him unfit for his responsibilities.

Jane Anne's family told me exactly what I needed to do in order to meet the state's educational requirements for teaching full time. Alabama A&M University, the Historically Black University in the area, offered a Master's in Education program, which I could complete in two years. Her parents also lined up a teacher's aide position in which I could work at the beginning of the next school year, while progressing toward obtaining my credentials to teach. For once in my life, everything was going like clockwork.

I stop by my grandmother's house on my way from working a leisurely third shift at the mall. I plan to eat a hearty breakfast at the ancient greasy spoon called simply, The Restaurant, where my cousin used to take me as a child. I had eaten there once or twice recently since rediscovering it. The coffee I never drank as a child is exquisite, and mixes so sweetly with the grease of the bacon. I walk into my grandmother's townhouse and everything is quiet, well lit, and well kept. I am still wearing my uniform, minus the ten-gallon hat. I walk up the stairs to my grandmother's room and I do not see Bert. When I see Grandmother, she is frightened out of her mind. Bert has done something that has frightened her. Something involving a BB gun and the neighbors, and other things she cannot comprehend.

When I go back downstairs, Bert is screaming uncontrollably. He is in a state of full uncontrollable psychosis. I cannot reason with him. I cannot communicate with him. I knew this would happen eventually. No one in the condition I had seen him in before could possibly remain stable for any length of time without treatment.

I telephone the police. He must go to the hospital now. A police officer finally arrives. The officer on the scene is someone I have never seen before. I can look into his eyes and see he is a genuine public servant, seasoned and true. He sees my uniform and does not see a loser trying to be a "rent a cop," but a young man trying to make his way through life.

I explain the situation to him, including my own mental illness, and how the quivering mass of emaciated flesh on the floor, who is somehow now managing to pull himself together just a little bit more at the sight of a police officer, is clearly having a psychotic break with reality. Bert is not able to get it together enough, though, for his answers to approach logical sense. Another police officer arrives and I do not even see his face, as the situation is causing me to lose focus. I do not even really hear the whole dialogue between Bert and the police. I am in a state of shock, and some part of me wants to maintain a sense of impartiality, despite the certain knowledge I have of my brother's situation. This is knowledge that hardly anyone has, since so very few people have experienced anything like this. This is like a scene from a living nightmare. The police question the neighbors. They question everybody. There is no question: Bert is going to the hospital.

I go upstairs and comfort Grandmother. She does not want Bert to come back to the house anymore. I try to explain to Grandmother what Bert is going through, but she is angry with him and does not seem to understand. Is it possible that she does not really understand what mental illness is all about? Even after all she has lived through, all she has lost. Has she become so elderly and physically frail that she has somehow forgotten all of this? Can she no longer relate to the world enough to see the obvious? The next time I sit on the couch downstairs it feels surreal. For years, I will have dreams of sitting on that couch and wondering, "Am I really here?" I thought I had been displaced from this house. Perhaps it was all a bad dream.

As Jane Anne and I prepared to visit my brother, Bert, at the behavioral medicine ward of Huntsville Hospital, I suspected that the fact that I had similar experiences and had even shared in those experiences with him almost two years before made me more understanding and compassionate to his situation than most brothers would be.

My girlfriend and I entered through the locked steel door that I had been through so many times before and signed in as visitors. We walked to my brother's room and saw him shackled to his bed with straps, ranting incoherently.

This unorthodox introduction was the first time Jane Anne had ever seen my brother, and she wore a shocked expression. This scene appeared strange to me, as well, as I had only seen people who had to be restrained a couple of times, and none of them were screaming as Bert was.

Bert's gaunt and unkempt appearance made the sight even more unusual. I felt guilty that my Jane Anne even had to witness this with me; I also felt a gnawing sense of unfairness at the fact that no one else was available to help me with this situation.

I filed a petition for my brother's commitment to a state hospital. There was no way I wanted him outside in his current state, and felt it was only right that he be given the same opportunity to come to grips with his mental illness that I had.

I filed the petition by going to the attorney's office who handled my own commitment proceeding not so long ago. The irony of the fact that I had been committed and was now filing a petition for my brother's commitment did not escape me. I was young to be placed in such a position of responsibility, but I was the only person available to handle this situation. One thing I learned while discussing this situation with the attorney was that by filing the petition, I ran the risk of having to pay for all of the court costs if I lost the case. This fact did not deter me, especially in light of the fact that Bert's case appeared like such a solid one. After a week passed, I entered the court alone to witness my brother's fate.

The same probate judge who had presided over my commitment was presiding. After hearing all of the evidence, and watching one of the police officers on the scene use the exact same trick as had been used on me by luring my brother into testifying on his own behalf, I sat on edge to hear the judge's decision. A deep sense of relief ran through me when the judge ruled that my brother would be committed to NARH.

Having looked at commitment proceedings for PLMI from both sides now, I must say that the probate court, in my view, is not at all typical of other kinds of court systems. The ruling to have my brother committed to a state institution was not, in fact, like sentencing a person to jail or prison, in that his sentence to the hospital was something that could only help him, and could not be seen in any way as a type of punishment.

Conversely, if Bert's defense attorney had been successful in defending him from losing his freedom temporarily, my brother might have been harmed and would have been sentenced to trying to manage symptoms of his mental illness without all of the help he needed.

These kinds of "mirror universe" court proceedings tend to make for a far less adversarial court system, where the court officers, including the judge, attorneys, and the person doing the psychological assessment usually agree.

Jane Anne went with me to visit my brother at the state hospital. Once while talking to him on the front steps, Bert and I began arguing over something minor. I became so frustrated that I began yelling at him and then at Jane Anne. The nurse on call, who was there when I was a patient, lowered his eyes, as if to say that I was losing control of my emotions. I was then able to regain my composure and apologize to them both.

I dutifully delivered my brother cigarettes, underwear, and whatever else my grandmother thought he needed while institutionalized. Like me, it took about two or three weeks for his psychotic symptoms to dissipate.

Bert remained in the hospital for about six weeks, as I had, and then he was placed in the group home, the same one I had lived in, until an apartment came available. I visited him at the group home, and had the surreal sensation of walking back in time through my own life and growth in the world of mental health. Bert would be living in the apartment across the hall from my own, we were told, and it was with great pride that I showed Bert around the complex. I described to Bert all of the different types of moves he would have to make, like applying for food stamps and for disability payments, in order to successfully survive in his new environment.

Just before Bert was scheduled to move to his apartment, he made a decision that seemed rather incomprehensible to me, but that he insisted upon, nonetheless. He told me that he would not be staying at the apartment, filing for disability, or doing any of the things that I was advising him to do. He said that he would instead find a way of making his life on his own without the assistance of the mental health system. He said that he could not accept the fact that he had a mental illness and didn't feel the need to live in a special program for PLMI. He also did not want to wait to file for disability payments, but wanted to start working right away.

"If I'm going to work and pay rent somewhere, why be forced to live here?" he asked.

I begged, pleaded, reasoned, and yelled for him to stay in the program. The mental health workers tried to convince Bert to continue in the program as well, but he signed his rights away to remain in Shelter Plus. Bert told me he had moved in with a friend of his in the neighboring town of Madison.

I knew Bert was making a bad decision, and the mental health staff knew he was making an awful decision; Bert, however, did not know how bad this decision was. I knew, though, that I had done everything in my power to help Bert receive the mental health assistance he needed. I could not live his life for him, though, and ultimately the decision was his to make.

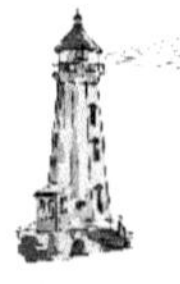

CENSUS BY DESIGN

In the summer of 2000, I was hired by the United States Census Bureau to work as an enumerator. I knew I had a job as a teacher's assistant waiting for me at the beginning of the next school year, since it had been guaranteed to me by school officials. Thinking that I no longer needed my security job at the mall, I informed by boss, Rick, that I would be resigning for the second time.

Since I was guaranteed a permanent job in the fall, it seemed to me like the natural course of action. My boss at the mall tried to explain the error of my decision. "Anything could happen, and this job is permanent, unlike the Census Bureau," he explained. Feeling confident about my plan, I paid him no heed and resigned anyway. I began my job with the Census Bureau enthusiastically, confident that I was finally moving on with my life.

Fate, I came to learn, can be a mistress who often has ideas of her own, and the next wave of family turmoil proved equally as daunting as the last.

My work with the Census Bureau was nearing its completion in August of 2000. I was told by my grandmother and stepfather, Dave, that he had made the decision to retire from his engineering job with the Department of the Army. After retiring, he would be moving to St. Louis, Missouri, to be near his son and daughter-in-law.

Dave was in his mid-seventies at this point and certainly well within all reasonable bounds to make this decision. Since he owned the house in which my grandmother lived, this meant that someone else would either have to take on the responsibility for the house payments, or else my grandmother would have to find somewhere else to live. My stepfather wrote a letter to my grandmother's brother who was an appellate judge in Texas. My stepfather was very forceful in his letter regarding his desire for my uncle to take some responsibility for my grandmother's care. The letter further stated that he would no longer be able to assume this responsibility himself.

The situation became more complicated when my girlfriend, who had ideas of marriage, actually telephoned my uncle's family, without my permission, to plead with them to help my grandmother in some way. I found it unacceptable that she would contact my uncle without speaking to me first. This led to angry words between us and we made the mutual decision to break up.

I took for granted the fact that I would not be taking on the teaching assistant's post in the fall after all, and I assumed further that my name would be "mud" in terms of ever finding a teacher's position in Madison County. This meant that my dreams of having a profession and a decent income were put on hold once more, and since I had quit my job at the mall and had no other income, I was back in the same old situation… unemployed.

My grandmother then received a letter from her brother stating that he had terminal cancer that had reached an advanced stage, and that he was not expected to live much longer. He further stated that he was not in a position to offer financial assistance. This left an air of gloom and sadness on everyone involved.

It was now up to me to try to sort things out as best I could, especially since my stepfather was still recovering from heart surgery, and I didn't want to burden him any more than necessary. I was in a balancing act. I had to try to meet the needs of my grandmother, my stepfather, and my own needs in as an efficient and orderly manner as possible.

After my responsibility for providing care and education for children had vanished, I stopped taking my medication for my psychiatric illness for a brief time. I went on a couple more job interviews in Tuscaloosa through the University's job placement program, and on one of those occasions I began to feel my mind unravel.

This was very different from previous psychotic experiences in that I clearly knew I had mental illness and understood clearly what to watch out for in terms of symptoms. What I experienced at that time may be described as a precursor to the types of psychotic symptoms I experienced before. My conscious mind refused to accept and believe the types of phenomena I was experiencing. Before, I had no knowledge of them as symptoms at all, and they were able to creep into all aspects of my mind before I knew what was happening to me.

What I remember most about this short-lived episode was that when I met my friend Rob at a barbecue restaurant in Birmingham, I could hardly concentrate on my conversation with him because it seemed that everyone in the restaurant was focusing their attention on me, and that all of their conversations were about me in some way. My head began to throb as I became extremely aware of everyone sitting in the restaurant, and it seemed in some way that they were all staring at me.

After we left the restaurant and were riding in Rob's car back to where he would drop me off, I told him of the types of sensations I was experiencing.

"I know it's clearly absurd, but it felt like everyone in that restaurant was focusing all their attention on me. It feels this way wherever I go, even though I tell myself it can't be possible and that it has to be a symptom of the illness I have. I've tried to tell myself that if I accept the fact that I have an illness, I could mentally prevent myself from experiencing anything like this, but now I see this isn't the case. I haven't been taking my medication for a while, and now it's clear that I have to do so; and hope that it takes these kinds of sensations out of my mind," I said.

Rob seemed to understand what I was telling him and agreed with my analysis. "I think you're right, Jim. Just get back on your medication when you get home."

I felt uncomfortable about the fact that we were even in a situation where I had to bounce these ideas off him, while also feeling grateful that he was there to hear me out. I made the drive back to Huntsville, which was indeed a rather difficult trip. Since the distracting psychotic experiences did not subside, I started back on my medication as soon as I got home. I was pleased to discover the symptoms subsided after a few days. Never again would I consider stopping my medication altogether, and I never experienced symptoms on that scale again. This was another crucial turning point. None of my future attempts to test my mental durability and stamina would ever involve the decision to neglect my prescribed medication for mental health.

I spent much time with my stepfather during this period, knowing that when he moved it would be unlikely that I would have enough money to pay for a trip to see him again for some time.

With Bert gone, we were now responsible for providing Grandmother's direct care ourselves. My stepfather and I took turns doing chores for her, and thankfully, we received an enormous amount of support in this area from a great number of people, including close family friends and neighbors.

Grandmother had aided so many of her older neighbors when I had been away at school, that many women now felt grateful for the opportunity to demonstrate their appreciation. Bert's presence, when he was unstable, had prevented much of this outpouring of aid from happening. We were all now working in concert to make Grandmother comfortable, until we could find somewhere else for her to live.

I told my therapist, Marilyn, that I was once more unemployed and was now required to assume additional responsibilities. "I think I should go ahead and file for disability payments," I said.

She said that I should have been receiving disability payments the entire time, and that I was unwise not to file for them as soon as they mysteriously vanished. I now saw the wisdom in her words and said, "I guess I should start back at Day Treatment," knowing I had to participate in some kind of structured activity in order to meet the guidelines of the Shelter Plus Program.

She then said something I didn't expect.

"Instead of attending Day Treatment, you could do volunteer work. I've lined up an interview for you at the local chapter of The National Alliance for the Mentally Ill."

The National Alliance for the Mentally Ill (now the National Alliance on Mental Illness (NAMI)) is a support and advocacy group for family members of people who have mental illness.

The NAMI Huntsville office was located in the United Way building. They had an extensive library containing information about mental health, as well as excellent facilities for people to meet and congregate. Volunteers were stationed by a telephone to answer the questions of anyone in need. NAMI was comprised of family members of PLMI, many of whom had spent much of their lives working to make lives better for people facing mental health issues. Most of the NAMI members were the parents of PLMI.

I found instant acceptance from members of NAMI, as well as great wisdom from their descriptions of their own experiences in trying to provide care for their family. I was invited to attend their meetings and became a member myself after explaining my failed attempts to try to help my brother to accept mental health care.

I learned that NAMI provided education to family members free of charge and were very learned and skilled in this matter. They even offered a training course called "Family to Family" which helped to prepare people for bearing the burden of having a loved one with mental illness. Hearing the experiences of other people helped me gain an even greater understanding of PLMI and their loved ones. We all had something in common in that we had all witnessed horrible difficulties in our families and were doing everything to make the best of the situation. I felt honored to be selected to work voluntarily for NAMI, and I was very thankful for the opportunity to learn more about myself, as well as others.

I went to Madison County's branch of the SSA, as well as to the DHR that authorized food stamps, in order to apply for a renewal of benefits. I knew that I was not capable of managing the family matters thrust upon me while finding and working a full-time job. My recent mental unraveling only bolstered my decision.

This time I did not enter the offices of SSA and DHR with the frightened eyes of a child newly learning that he has been diagnosed with a lifelong degenerative illness—rather with the eyes of a person with a polite, but matter-of-fact attitude. I knew that I was eligible for these benefits and that the support of my family depended upon them, and I was not willing to let either them or myself down. I filled out the paperwork for disability insurance on my own this time, and waited for a response.

I learned through my therapist that there was an agency in place whose purpose was to help people in my grandmother's situation, as well as their families. I went to the Area Agency on Aging and spoke to a woman who was an ombudsman. This ombudsman's position was created to consult with families that had aging parents, like my own. The ombudsman set up an appointment for me and my stepfather to see an agency attorney free of charge. We met with the attorney who spoke to us about our options for my grandmother, Colice.

The attorney was a kind black woman recently out of law school. She asked us questions about Grandmother's assets, and upon hearing that she had none, told us that Colice would have to be hospitalized for three days before she could be accepted to a nursing home.

I also enlisted the aid of Bill, my adopted brother's mother, whose name was Betty. Betty was a nurse, and she drove me around to see some different nursing homes. She helped me explain my family's situation to the homes and to ask about the possibility for placement. A home called Windsor House seemed interested in taking Grandmother Colice in, and it came to be my grandmother's home for the remaining years of her life.

Windsor House had once been one of the city's two hospitals, and I became very familiar with its halls before my association with it was completed. My stepfather visited the home with me, and we agreed that Grandmother would be comfortable there. My grandmother had to be hospitalized for three days before she could be admitted, but she resisted. But we called an ambulance and coaxed her into going to the hospital with them for the mandatory three days.

I was there when my grandmother was first admitted to Windsor House. She was very scared and almost in a state of shock when she arrived. The nursing home staff and I did all we could to comfort her, and after a couple of days, she seemed much more adjusted to the idea, and became calmer.

While all this was in process, I visited my stepfather frequently and discussed plans for his, and my own, future. I still owed a great deal of money for hospital bills, as well as other debt. "Maybe it would be good for you to look into bankruptcy," he said. His son, Wendell, happened to be a bankruptcy attorney and he encouraged me strongly to speak to him.

When I spoke to Wendell, he told me that I should file chapter seven bankruptcy, otherwise known as a "straight seven," and should speak to an attorney right away for this purpose. I went to an attorney my stepfather recommended through his own attorney. He was about five years older than me and wore wire-frame glasses.

The fact that it had been my goal to have the same position as his, and that I was now in the situation in which I found myself, was not lost on either of us. The attorney said that the process would cost about seven hundred dollars, half of which I could pay at the beginning. Dave put up the money to get the process underway.

While I waited for a response from the SSA, something rather curious happened. The SSA sent the same forms I had spent a great deal of time completing already and asked me to fill them out all over again. I had not thought to make copies of these forms, and had to start over in order to fill them out. This made absolutely no sense to me, but I suspected it was a way to try to prevent people from applying for disability benefits.

Determined not to fill out the same forms over repeatedly for an indefinite period, I called my bankruptcy lawyer and asked him to refer me to another lawyer who could help me to handle my disability case. He directed me to an attorney who was happy to take my case, and left me with the impression that it would be a simple matter for him to win. The three attorneys who had helped me tremendously in these family matters from my grandmother's care, to bankruptcy, to disability all left me with the indelible impression that there were a number of legal professionals in the country who were using their considerable abilities to help people just like me. If my fate had been one in which I myself had become an attorney, I hope I would have utilized my position to help people in need like these people helped me.

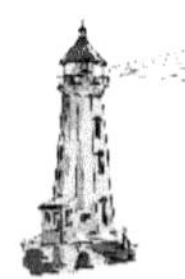

NEW FRONTIER

I'm standing in the Extraterrestrial Museum in Roswell New Mexico, the town where aliens reportedly crash landed in 1947. On the walls I see enlarged newspaper clippings touting the arrival of these aliens. On the floor there are child-sized stuffed dummies with enlarged heads and eyes with fluorescent green skin, wearing silver space suits. For some reason I am not as impressed with the museum, as I thought I might be prior to entering.

Perhaps it's because my hometown of Huntsville, Alabama features an amazing Space and Rocket Center, on acres of ground, replete with giant models of rockets of all varieties, including the Saturn V that made it to the moon, as well as the Space Shuttle. As a child I often went on field trips to the Space and Rocket Center and remember eyeing the innards of various human-made spaceships and space gear of all varieties.

One of the most memorable exhibits there for me was the glass cage which housed the most famous squirrel monkey in human history. Mrs. Baker was the first American life form to travel from earth into space. The Russians sent the first life form from earth, which happened to be a dog. Mrs. Baker also had a male companion that lived in the glass cage with her to keep her company. This companion, or husband, as some referred to him, outlived Mrs. Baker by many years, and continued to remain on exhibit for children to visit after her death.

On the way to Roswell, New Mexico, we rode past the Very Large Array of huge radio telescopes pointing toward the cosmos to discover whatever it may. We stopped at an empty museum-like building there which had information about the Very Large Array and its history.

I can't help but think about the large satellite dishes that I helped to construct between the ages of ten and twelve in rural areas through Alabama while spending summers with one of the families who helped to raise me, who just happened to own a small satellite dish installation business.

Business was booming at that time as people raced to purchase these dishes, which could pull cable television of all varieties for free out of the thin air. When the cable channel companies figured out a way to scramble the signals such that people then had to rent descrambling devices to watch them, the family's business was lost in fairly short order.

As a child though, my small frame made me uniquely suited to certain tasks, such as lying underneath the dishes with a wrench so that others could screw the four sections of the dishes together. Many years later, dishes would become much smaller in size due to technological advancements. My size had also made it easy for me to crawl underneath houses in order to feed the wires up to the adults above the floor. I learned almost nothing about the actual technology and wiring inherent in the complicated technological devices, though, either because of my age or a lack of inclination—most probably both.

While in Roswell, we sleep in a school gymnasium, as we do in so many of the small towns we ride through. Like the other small towns we stop in, I can't help but be enamored with this one. I find the emptiness of the streets compelling somehow as I wander through them. Perhaps being born and mostly raised in a medium-sized city has something to do with this sense of charm inspired by small towns. After Roswell we'll pass through the towns of West Texas, and in particular the town of Lubbock, which I will be completely enthralled with for the rest of my life. I'll go to a gigantic line-dancing hall there filled with people, many with cowboy hats and all with boots, and I'll think it's one of the coolest things I've ever seen. Similar gatherings packed to the gills with people listening to country music will be etched into my memory. I'll even visit a shop that sells used boots and purchase a pair for ten dollars, which I find amazing.

For now though, I remain in the E.T. museum musing on the events which occurred nearly fifty years ago in that small area in New Mexico. I always argued with extended family members that extraterrestrials of some form or another have to be real because mathematically, it would make no sense for them not to be. I also spend much of my youth watching science fiction movies and television shows, as well as collecting comic books, which likely shaped my views in this area to a large degree. An Italian philosopher named Giordano Bruno was burned at the stake, in 1600, for claiming that there are multiple worlds, some of which may be home to sentient beings of their own. My views are not condemned to that degree by the general population of the mid nineteen nineties, yet they are certainly not seen as mainstream either. I exit the tiny tourist trap thankful for my memories there and ready to continue my Journey of Hope to places new to me.

I had been transformed by my experiences of the past four years. My ability and luck in weathering these experiences had propelled me into a position of some distinction and inspiration to those who found themselves within the world of mental health. But to all outside observers, I was merely an unemployed man who had a mental illness.

Few people, then and today, know much about mental diseases or, more specifically, schizophrenia. While I was becoming reasonably more comfortable in my own skin and beginning to accept my situation, I continued to be highly self-conscious about my mental health status, particularly around people who weren't part of the mental health community.

Part of the metamorphosis I underwent at that time included my decision to quit drinking alcohol. I had spent many periods of time in the past four years often drinking to excess. This behavior, I decided, was unwise, considering my situation. Alcohol and psychotropic medications definitely do not mix and can lead to severe and destructive consequences.

On the one hand, I felt very fortunate to have endured the decision-making process regarding my family, without breaking down completely. On the other hand, I felt like I had failed in many ways to make my life what I, and those who knew me, thought it could be. I certainly thought that I would be perceived as something of a failure to those who did not know I had a mental illness.

I decided to go to my stepfather's house to speak with him about family business, to an extent, but primarily about life in general. "Do you want something to drink? I have water or wine," he offered.

"I don't drink alcohol, anymore," was my reply. He just looked at me curiously and shrugged.

I sat in his cluttered living room and he showed me a new object of interest. It was a Roman Pilum that he crafted, by hand. The Roman Pilum was a type of spear that could be thrown at enemy infantry. It made a fine addition to his household, which was a museum of all kinds of novelties, like model trains and airplanes, as well as an arsenal of weaponry from innumerable wars and conflicts throughout history.

I would miss this man greatly after his move to St. Louis, but I didn't comprehend this fully while he sat in front of me with a smile on his face. We were grateful to each other for the efforts we'd made to safeguard my grandmother's health the best we could. I expected to receive my disability payments any day, and was surviving on food stamps and my apartment program, which allowed me to live rent-free while I had no income. I told my stepfather that the bankruptcy I filed was well under way and that I was awaiting my day in court for that purpose. I described to him how my main source of entertainment was reading books and watching movies checked out of the library to supplement basic cable provided by my apartment. On my way out, Dave said, "Most of the things I enjoy cost relatively little money, anyway."

I returned to my apartment. It felt good to plop on my couch and enjoy watching television and reading without having to worry about where I was going to get my next meal. The memories I had of barely being able to read a paragraph seemed to fade into the distant mists of memory. I only had to do my volunteer job once every two weeks and had all the time in the world. I loved to watch Judge Mathis on television every day.

I visited my grandmother at least once a week and we spoke about anything on our minds. In this sense, I felt like the luckiest man on the planet; I got to see the woman who was my closest companion as often as I wished. She had access to a cadre of caregivers and round-the-clock health care at Windsor house. It did not take her long to realize that she was much better off in this new environment than she had been in the confines of her room at the townhouse.

There was now no one in my apartment complex that I was extremely close to. There were perhaps five or six residents of the complex that I visited on occasion or had a brief conversation with while passing by.

One of those people was an elderly woman who lived downstairs, with whom I shared a cup of coffee from time to time, and who I gave rides to whenever she needed them. Ruth was part of the smoking circle I had joined when I first arrived at the apartment complex. She had the habit of asking me to drive her to the same pawn-shop, where she pawned the same television set at least once every other month. She would not accept a loan from me as she thought it would somehow damage our neighborly friendship. I ended up providing transportation for a number of my neighbors, when they requested it. They all paid me a few dollars for gas.

I wished desperately to form a new romantic relationship. It was painfully obvious to me that this was nowhere on the horizon. I telephoned Karen, my friend in Birmingham, and told her that I had a mental illness and that I was doing volunteer work. I never heard from her again. I was no longer surprised by this outcome, though it was no easier for me to bear. I tended to isolate myself, not knowing where to turn for friends or sweethearts.

The members of NAMI tended to be older than I, and while I enjoyed their company, there were no romantic prospects developing for me there. I remained thankful that life events had gone as well as they had, although there was a noticeable void in my life, in terms of personal fulfillment, that would continue for some time.

By November of 2000, I began receiving disability payments. The only major change I made to my lifestyle was in purchasing a new car. I had several thousand dollars left over after I paid nine hundred dollars to my disability lawyer.

I bought a green 1992 Buick Le Sabre that was fully loaded. It was, by far, the nicest car I had ever owned, and I proudly showed it off to my stepfather who, with a smile on his face, complimented me. He had always bought old, very inexpensive economy cars, and did all mechanical repairs to them himself. Unfortunately, I did not learn this skill and was subject to the whims of fate regarding car maintenance.

The family, consisting of my grandmother, my stepfather, me, and Bert, did not spend Christmas together for the first time in sixteen years, but I did receive about five hundred dollars from my stepfather.

Grandmother handed the wad of cash to me, and I knew instinctively that this money must have come from his sale from many of my grandmother's possessions I had refused to save.

A few of the possessions, like a coffee table and my grandmother's bed, I was able to place in a storage room maintained by my brother, David, who had filed the petition on me three years before. The other items I had no idea what to do with, and in many ways, I felt a mental block about trying to figure out what to do with them.

Many of my reservations about handling these furnishings had to do with memories of Bert destroying some of her most prized valuables while he was living with Grandmother in a psychotic state. I had been helpless to do anything about the destruction.

In one instance, there were ancient copies of William Shakespeare's *The Merchant of Venice* and *Romeo and Juliet* enclosed in a glass frame. Grandmother had told me since I was a young child that these would belong to me whenever she passed on. Bert had taken these antique manuscripts out of the glass case and had ripped them apart in order to create some kind of collage that had coalesced in his imbalanced mind.

My grandmother and I spent her first Christmas at Windsor House, by ourselves, in her room. This felt like a solemn occasion, in many respects, tinged with pure love as well as with vibrant sorrow. We discussed past Christmases, while we enjoyed the present one together. Grandmother was particularly sad about the loss of her brother, who had passed away from cancer a few months ago.

My grandmother had much to do with his upbringing, and my jealousy of the affection she gave him left me unable to offer the proper empathy for her loss. She told me that I should really be more understanding of what she was experiencing, and I made a mental note to try to be more appreciative of her situation. I had not learned that her sorrow was her own, and that it was not my place to judge how she expressed it. I managed to learn this lesson quickly, though, and reached the conclusion that I should merely listen to her express her sadness, and not try to encourage her to simply look on the bright side of things.

Thanks to receiving disability payments again, I had some money, and I decided to try to resume socializing at bars, but this time on my own terms, as a non-drinker. I discovered that I am one of the very few people who can, in fact, "hang out" in bars without drinking alcohol, but I was unable to sustain this socializing for other reasons that had nothing to do with alcohol.

Not only did I not have a job, but also many of the people at the local bar I frequented knew by this time that I had a mental illness. This created something of a noticeable barrier between us. Meeting new people created complications, as well, in the sense that the first question that they always seemed to ask was, "What do you do?" When I would tell them that I was a volunteer worker at the local chapter of NAMI, a number of awkward questions would arise.

I also found that I really did not have much in common with the other bar patrons, other than a desire to meet women. I never fully penetrated into the social circles of those who spent time in the bars, even during the times when I was employed or had some known prospect for my future. After a month of pursuing socialization in this arena, I gave it up, choosing to be isolated in my apartment.

The time for my stepfather to make his move to St. Louis came closer. This move didn't take place with much fanfare, since I spent much of my time trying to avoid him during his final months in Huntsville because of my reluctance to try to figure out what to do with my grandmother's possessions, which he had stored in his house.

When leaving his house the last time I saw him, he had left some large clippers in the yard that he was trying to sell. I went to return the clippers to him, walking quickly. When I got to the small step outside his door, he was speeding out to return the sunglasses that I had accidentally left in his chair.

He had a look of urgency on his face as he sped out the door and called my name not realizing that I had returned with the clippers. If I had not been holding the blades face down as he had taught me as a small child when handling the clippers, he might have stood a real chance of impaling himself on them in his haste to see me one more time.

We looked into one another's eyes as we both realized simultaneously what neither one of us could really put into words—we shared a strong bond, but him not being able to live a life of freedom, untethered by my family and its needs, was killing him. I now had only the knowledge he helped to create in me to make my way through life, on my own. I would have to employ the lessons he and others taught me in order to avoid the inevitable collision with life that could ruin us. He had grown old and must see to his own needs, while I was still young and must make my own way the best I could. Any deviation from this pattern could be destructive to us both.

This was another one of his valuable lessons. Sometimes you have to remove yourself from a situation that is causing unbearable stress, even if it causes some pain to yourself and others. We nodded to each other as I processed this analogy with a look of hopeful pride on my face. His eyes showed resigned sadness.

UNTITLED MELODY

In April 2001, I attended the annual Consumer Conference in Shocco Springs for a second time. I enjoyed the conference again, especially because I was even more accepting of myself as someone living with schizophrenia. I had been taking medication on my own for almost an entire year and felt well-versed in what it took to stay in recovery from serious mental illness.

The conference was eventful, as always, and it was great to see the attendees there. The sun was really beating down on me, and I was becoming very stimulated by the throng of people and the conversation.

Then, something very curious happened. My mind began to feel like it was sort of fading out, for lack of a better description. This was unlike any symptom I had experienced before this time. It was as if I could not focus on any one thing. I was not imagining things without evidence, or seeing or hearing things that were not there, but I lost practically all ability to concentrate. Furthermore, I was trembling noticeably and could not seem to stop. My ability to converse fled me as I fearfully tried to grasp what was happening to me. I did not even consider trying to consult professional help at that point, thinking that whatever was happening would end soon. With the conference completed, I made a dash for my car and drove home using all of the focus I could muster.

By the time I arrived at my apartment, I discovered that I continued to feel just as badly as I had since the beginning of my spell, if not worse. I thought that in the confines of my apartment, whatever was happening to me would end instantaneously, and was horrified when I discovered that it did not.

When I tried to watch television, it seemed to be a blaring trumpet that I couldn't concentrate on in the least. I had somewhat programmed myself to resist any thoughts about going to the hospital, since I knew it was a last resort, but I thought that it might be what I should do if I could not figure out anything else. Panicking further, I telephoned my stepfather and reported to him what I was experiencing.

"I'm fading out. I can't focus on anything. I thought I had it all together, but I can't even read the words I'm trying to read now. They seem like only a blur. My vision is phasing in and out and I'm shaking like a leaf," I said.

Dave then said words which, though very simple, had great power and calming resonance.

"Your brain is like the engine in your car. You must take care of it the same way you do that machine. You have to be careful about putting too much stress or strain on it. You must make sure it has everything it requires; the same way you would make sure your car engine has oil and water," he said.

We said our goodbyes, and although my stepfather's words did not solve my immediate problem, they did make a lasting impression on me, in terms of conceptualizing my brain in a mechanistic way. Like any other organ, such as the heart or the lungs, my brain operated according to certain physical laws, which I made every effort to understand.

I knew I had to seek aid elsewhere, or else I would certainly have to make an appearance at the hospital, breaking the two-year period of time I had managed to keep from being admitted. My fear of going back into debt fueled my resolve to stay out of the hospital as much as anything else.

I walked over to one of my neighbor's apartments and spoke to the man who lived there, explaining what happened. He was a white-haired black man, named Max, who had been in recovery from his mental illness for a long time. When he was struck with his mental illness, he had been married with children, working in cable television installation.

I explained to him what I was experiencing and asked him what was happening, and if I should go to the hospital.

"Have you been out in the sun for a long time," he asked. "Yes, I have," I answered.

He then told me that this had likely caused an adverse reaction to my medication. Suddenly all the admonitions the women affectionately termed, "NAMI Mommies" had given me about being out in the sun for too long came rushing into my mind. Who could believe that sitting out in the sun for a long time could cause me to experience all of this?

Max said, "You need to lie down in your apartment in the dark and cool for a while. Drink plenty of cool water, and don't watch TV or listen to the radio."

I went to my apartment and did exactly as he had told me. After a couple of days lying in my bed, I began to feel much better, and was extremely thankful. I had learned a new skill. By listening to the advice of my friend, I had effectively turned my own home into a personal hospital, and avoided having to be admitted to another facility. I could deal with many serious problems without having to lose my personal freedom or taking up valuable resources.

The thought occurred to me that I had become so different a person that I had to think about such things, such as how long I could endure sunlight. Occurrences like this transcended factors such as gender, age, and race to create a powerful bond between PLMI. When my neighbor helped me to cope with the reaction of sunlight with my medication, our differences in skin color was not nearly as important as our similarities in brain chemistry were.

My stepfather made his move to Missouri, and we stopped communicating for a time. He wrote letters to my grandmother periodically, which I read to her. I made no effort to contact him during this period.

In part, I felt ashamed of what I was, and what I was not, and I couldn't face my shame in talking to him. It didn't occur to me at that time that it might hurt his feelings that I didn't make more of an effort to contact him. It did occur to me that he was making no effort to contact me, either, other than in the form of letters written to Grandmother, and I thought that it might cause him unnecessary stress to have to speak to me; and I certainly didn't want that.

Around the time of my grandmother's move to her new home, a new person became a fixture in our lives. She was a distant family relation, in her fifties, who I will call Samantha. She and her husband lived in Huntsville and were quite wealthy. Like Grandmother, who had provided care for ill family members throughout her lifetime, Samantha was well-versed at caring for people. She and her husband were members of the church where I had caused the scene described earlier.

From the time Grandmother moved to Windsor House, Samantha took a serious interest in her well-being. She visited Grandmother regularly, and showered her with attention, gifts, and loving care. She did not take any particular interest in me, except as someone who was part of my grandmother's life. This was something of a new phenomenon for me, as in all of my experience, anyone in my or Grandmother's life seemed to take great interest in the both of us or in me.

It became immediately clear that she was going to be a rival for my grandmother's affection. I saw instantly that she could provide resources with which I could not compete. I then became unhappily aware of what my grandmother must have experienced throughout my childhood. Many families took interest in my well-being, and she must have often felt what I was experiencing now, without the ability or resources to provide many of the things that these families could.

Grandmother's skill at negotiating these relationships was superb, and the instincts I must have picked up from her, surfaced without hesitation, causing me to immediately resist any impulse to push this rival away. I would not interfere in her care, but merely continue to play my role in my grandmother's new life in every way possible. Inevitably, a very strong bond was formed between Grandmother and my rival, Samantha, that was as strong as the bond between Grandmother and me, and I couldn't do anything to disrupt it without risking a diminishment in my grandmother's quality of life.

My grandmother's friend, Samantha, had both the know-how to see to my grandmother's needs as well as the clout to keep the nursing home on its toes. I had to honor the effectiveness with which my grandmother saw to my upbringing by emulating the diligence with which she cared for me.

I admired this woman's compassion and commitment to humanity for the care she provided my grandmother, even to the point where I feel I owe her an enormous and perhaps un-payable debt. The fact that she did not really seem to me to be completely empathetic to my situation is unfortunate, but rather insignificant to the grand scheme of things concerning my family as a whole.

My feelings of insignificance in this lady's opinion was more palpable and difficult for me to understand since I was surrounded by other people close to her age, at the NAMI and at the HMCMHC, who seemed always to express thoughts of warmth and admiration for me.

My grandmother was the most charming woman that I, and most everyone else, knew. Her enormous capacity to cope with life's tragedies only added to her mystique. Samantha tended to look upon me as someone who was not worthy of Grandmother Colice's love and devotion.

Once again, it is only an extremely exceptional person who takes on this kind of a job. But the personal strength that this new person in our lives had, which made her so capable of providing loving care to Grandmother, did not extend to treating me with anything but the barest courtesy.

This new relationship probably drew me even closer to the families of NAMI and the staff who cared for me at the HMCMHC. My involvement with NAMI gave me opportunities for involvement in the mental health community that I was quick to seize upon when opportunities were available. I attended NAMI conferences throughout the state, for instance, which NAMI Huntsville paid for. These conferences added to my knowledge and strengthened my feeling of communion with the family members of PLMI.

At the United Way building, I had access to the staff of the Mental Health Association (MHA), which was located in an office down the hall from NAMI. The MHA was a national organization whose primary purpose was to provide information to the community at large about various mental health issues.

The new popular understanding of depression and its prevalence, for instance, is due in large measure to the efforts of MHA campaigns to enhance public understanding of the illness. Another feature of the MHA, which was highly important, was the social gatherings that they put together for PLMI.

In Huntsville, these weekly gatherings are known as the Aquarius Club, and feature bingo, great food, and fellowship. A variety of guest speakers are invited to speak to the PLMI at these gatherings, as well. I took great pleasure in participating in these events, since they were a regular part of Day Treatment, when I attended it.

The director of the MHA when I worked at NAMI was a man

named Todd Cannon. I enjoyed talking with him from time to time when I was at the office, and on one occasion accepted his invitation to speak to a group of women at a civic function about what it was like to live with a mental illness.

Mental illness is not something that is immediately recognizable in someone, and the women I spoke to at the function seemed surprised that a seemingly healthy young man was among the ranks of those with mental illness.

I did my best to describe my situation to them, including the types of symptoms I had experienced. They wanted to know how I paid my bills, and I told them that I received disability insurance as my means of income. They wanted to know why I didn't have a job, and I found myself explaining to them many of the realities of my situation. I explained to them that I had to take daily medication that costs over three hundred dollars per month. I also told them that I wasn't in a position to find a job with insurance that could pay for these medications at this time in my life, and that in a job without insurance I would be at risk of losing the health benefits I already had.

I explained this catch-22 to them as best I could, and concluded that it would be unreasonable for me, or anyone in my position, to risk their mental health by putting themselves in a situation which would clearly be even more undesirable than the one in which they already found themselves. I did not go out of my way to speak of the family difficulties that had further hindered my efforts to improve my situation, but I did my best to keep within the boundaries of describing the situations of all PLMI.

I maintained my position on the Consumer Council at the HMCMHC and accepted the invitation from Louis, the man who had driven me to my first Consumer Conference, to attend the Manic-Depressive Support Group. Louis had been the president of this group that had met once a month at the HMCMHC for approximately thirty years. I explained to Louis that I did not have a diagnosis of depression, though I had experienced lows that had to be on a par with depressive symptoms, and he assured me that I was welcome in any case.

Schizophrenia has a set of symptoms, known as negative symptoms, which take away energy and initiative and cause a depressed mood. Additionally, there is a phenomenon known as post-psychotic depression which often occurs immediately after one has experienced a psychotic break with reality. Doubtless, there are chemical as well as situational issues that cause these symptoms to occur. I had been in the throes of all these factors in varying degrees ever since I had received my initial diagnosis in 1996, and I could easily identify with those who experienced depressive symptoms.

The attendees of these meetings were all clients of the HMCMHC, and they had varied levels of cognitive functioning. Louis was adept at facilitating the group discussion that took place, and at addressing everyone's concerns.

It was at this meeting that I met a middle-aged woman who was new to working at the HMCMHC and had been asked to represent the staff at the Manic-Depressive Support Group. Bernice was very personable and seemed to have a natural rapport with all of the clients. It was shortly after this meeting that Marilyn, who had been my therapist for the past four years, informed me that my case would be transferred to another therapist; and as it turned out, it was to be Bernice.

Marilyn, had been with me throughout that initial tumultuous four-year period of my life, and it was no small change for me to be transferred to a new therapist. She explained to me that insurance considerations had led to my transfer. I had worked at paid jobs so much that I now had two forms of health insurance, Medicaid and Medicare. I now had to see a therapist who was a Medicare provider.

Although I missed seeing Marilyn, who had been such an important part of my life, I developed an instant rapport with Bernice, who was very approachable. Bernice was in her early fifties with short brown hair, and it was apparent that she had a tremendous amount of experience as a therapist. We met at an entirely different phase of my growth as a PLMI, and our sessions were very different in nature from the ones I had with Marilyn.

My primary mission had ceased being a constant desire to figure out what I was going to do to survive and form a career, but now was more focused on how I could maintain my current state of mental health and make baby steps toward a future. I understood now that I was eligible to receive Social Security Disability benefits, and that it was perfectly understandable for me to receive these benefits for as long as I needed them.

Bernice and I were on the same “wavelength” with this, and she never put any excess stress upon me with regard to getting a job. At the same time, she had an instinct for nudging me out of my complacency whenever she could. While Marilyn had done an excellent job of explaining to me that I was being harder on myself than I would be to another person in the same situation, Bernice stressed that I had to be who I was and had to be comfortable with myself while doing so.

SUBMARINE IN SHADES OF GREY

I'm in a Civil War battleground memorial in Mississippi that we've bicycled to, and the number of graves around me seems endless. I don't realize this now, but I will see similar memorial gravesites in my distant future. One of these will be Arlington Cemetery in Washington D.C. in 2010. Another will be part of the Veteran's Administration, Illiana, in 2017, where I will work for a time, in a town called Danville, in Central Illinois. While in Illinois, I will also visit Abraham Lincoln's tomb, located in a large cemetery in the capitol city of Springfield. Standing in front of the black sarcophagus, I feel as if I'm being pulled into some kind of vortex. I ask myself if this feeling is being caused by my knowledge of the symbolism surrounding this situation or by something else even more profound. President Lincoln's promise to veterans, which is the V.A.'s official motto, is, "To care for him who shall have born the battle, and for his widow, and his orphan." I certainly feel fortunate to have the opportunity to do just that.

My apartment, in Danville, is located two blocks away from the home of Abraham Lincoln's bodyguard, who was a man named Ward Hill Lamon. During a festival featuring an enormous car show in the surrounding park, I will go inside this house and bear witness to people reenacting the lives of the people who lived in this home in the 1800's. They own an iron oven, of a sort, that was considered a very modern convenience for that time. A couple of years from then, I will see a movie based on the life of that man, called Saving Lincoln, *and learn about he and the sixteenth president's relationship in greater detail. This is the first feature film to utilize CineCollage technology to merge actors and set props with actual period photographs. This process helped to create a movie which was educational and visually compelling.*

Back in Mississippi, now I'm looking at an ironside ship and a sign describing its imperviousness to enemy shells. "You know at one point, the South even had a bicycle-powered submarine," I hear someone say. I think to myself, "what could be worse for our country than another civil war?"

At a point in my life when I felt largely ostracized by people who were not a part of the mental health community, Bernice did much to help me see the positive aspects of my life and helped me maintain my ability to count my blessings.

Counting my blessings came easier with the addition of a new neighbor, who in many ways was struggling more than I was. He had come to the Shelter Plus housing program in a rather circuitous way. A program reaching out to the city's homeless population had taken an interest in him, and helped him get a place in the apartment program. He explained that the program was now defunct due to lack of funding, but had managed to find him housing before going under. Although I felt a tinge of pain because of the fact that he was moving into the apartment that I hoped my brother would move into, I did everything I could to make him feel welcome, and we became friends.

The man, whom I will call Jeff, was an Army veteran, and I learned that when he revealed that he was ineligible to receive any medical services from the HMCMHC; he would have to travel all the way to the Veterans Admiration Medical Center, in Birmingham, one-hundred miles away, to receive any medical care, mental or physical. He was used to living in missions, and as it turned out, he was acquainted with my brother, Bert.

He was reed-thin, and years of hard living were etched onto his pale face. His balding, curly red hair was often concealed by a cap. He had a serious alcohol and drug addiction, from which he was trying to recover. He attended Narcotics Anonymous religiously and would go through stages in which he would rail out against all people who abused substances of any sort.

I learned valuable lessons from this man about people with addictions, and watched, in surprise, as he would stand on his balcony and seem to see people involved in drugs everywhere; sometimes he would even yell in rage at people passing by.

I asked him why he did not simply live and let live, deducing logically that there was likely to be drug use in every neighborhood in

America. He had no good answer for me but merely shook his head, as if the very notion of drugs was an affront to his inner being. He had no income, collected food stamps, and was filing for disability, with little success.

We shared information regarding survival, and dealt with the incessant barrage of the loneliness in our lives by talking to each other. His struggle to survive was much more difficult than mine because he was caught in a situation in which he could not work at all. If he worked, he would instantly become ineligible to receive disability income. His mental illness, however, was considered much less severe than mine, and he doubted he would be granted disability insurance payments at all.

One way Jeff survived was by selling his blood, at least twice a week. I was always in need of extra cash and I decided to try it.

This turned out to be a more intense experience than I could have ever bargained for, from the start to the end. I drove Jeff to a place called the plasma bank and prepared myself to "step on up to the plate."

First, I had to fill out forms to determine my eligibility to be a plasma donor. The forms asked questions such as if I had any illnesses such as HIV/AIDS or Hepatitis, and asked a number of questions to see if I was at risk of any of these illnesses. I answered "no" to them. The questionnaire also asked me to list any medications I took. Next, I went through an interview process with a woman who must have been nineteen or twenty. I was twenty-six years old.

I assumed the interview would be a rather simple process. I was wrong, as I found out very shortly into the interview. I answered the woman's questions in a very polite and succinct manner, since she asked them in a rather brisk way, revealing the irritation she had at having to ask any of these questions at all. When she asked me why I took Seroquel daily, I told her it was for a mental illness. She then began questioning me intensively about what metal illness I had, what symptoms I had and so forth.

I then asked her, trying to contain my obvious discomfort, "What does my having a mental illness have to do with any of this?"

She snapped in an angry tone, "I have to make sure that you don't do anything wild, like thinking you need to pull the tubes out of your arm, and having the blood go everywhere."

She then gestured to me in a way that seemed to imply that I should realize this, when in fact, no thought like this had ever even occurred to me. I figured my calm manner and deliberate speech would clearly dispel any notions of this sort that she might have had, but I was obviously mistaken. I assured her that I had no intention of creating a problem, and watched as she assented grudgingly to me selling blood plasma. I sat on a gurney surrounded by about twenty other people, mostly younger than me, as they drew blood from my arm.

I visited my grandmother at the nursing home the next day and told her that I had sold some of my blood, and that it had made me nauseous. She didn't have the reaction that I expected her to have about this fact, and seemed aghast at the very notion that I would sell my blood. I told her that it did not seem like such a bad idea at the time, and she told me not to ever do it again, especially since I had become as sick as I had. I assured her that I wouldn't.

My friend, Jeff, on the other hand, continued to sell his blood regularly, counting on it as his primary source of income. He shrugged away my decision not to do so anymore.

Crisis reared its ugly head in my life to some smaller degree as a kind of aftershock to what I had experienced in the past. One day, I received a telephone call from the man my brother moved in with after he left the Group Home. Bert had lived with a man named Hubey on and off over the years, and the man was fairly familiar with Bert's quirks. The man said in a panicked voice that Bert was exhibiting frightening symptoms that he had never seen before, and he did not know what to do.

This was the first time I remember speaking to Hubey, but I knew that Grandmother had spoken to him on many occasions. I told him of my experiences related to Bert's commitment and informed him of his options.

A couple of weeks later, while I was watching television in my apartment, my neighbor, Jeff, who knew my brother, told me that something was going on with Bert at one of the gas stations down the street from the apartment complex.

One of the rescue missions that housed the homeless was also located just down the street. I raced to the gas station to see what was happening, thinking that Bert might have moved into the mission. When

I arrived on the scene at the gas station, Bert was in a state of complete psychosis and was writhing on the ground screaming, surrounded by police officers. An ambulance transported Bert to the hospital in short order.

Another petition was then filed for my brother's commitment. This time the probate judge who had presided over so many of the important events in my life, from my adoption, to my own commitment, to the commitment of my brother, was preparing to retire, and I was informed that the hearing would be presided over by the new probate judge.

It was at this time that I discovered that the person wearing the black robe of the probate judge does not have to be an attorney at all, but can in fact be any citizen of Madison County. The new man elected to preside over the probate court was another official in the courthouse establishment, though not an attorney.

I prepared for the hearing by meeting the man who was Bert's roommate through so many periods of his life, in person, for the first and only time. Hubey described Bert's mental decline which had led to him having to ask my brother to leave his house.

Hubey was clueless with regard to the commitment process, and I did my best to prepare him for what to expect while listening to his description of Bert's symptoms. We went to the probate hearing and I was surprised when the court clerk told me that the retiring probate judge would be presiding over the court for this hearing. Once again, the symptoms my brother had been experiencing were based very much on religion, and the nature of freedom of religion was called into question.

Bert had been yelling delusional statements to the non-existent entities that he believed were attempting to take over his soul. He would yell out "I said no!" and "begone!" to the evil spirits he perceived. These did not warrant Bert's commitment to the hospital, in the eyes of the law, since they did not pose a danger to himself or other people. My brother was so gaunt that his ribs were poking out because he had eaten almost nothing for weeks in his religious fervor to observe the practice of fasting from food.

My brother was finally ruled to be mentally incompetent because his refusal to eat was deemed to be a danger to himself. This time it was determined that he didn't have to be sent to the state hospital. Instead he would be committed to the group home for a time. He would be subject to commitment to the state hospital if he refused to stay in the group home, as ordered.

Bert followed through with his commitment to the group home, where I visited him regularly. I was surprised to learn that he had even met a girlfriend while living there. Unfortunately, his commitment to trying to live life outside the mental health system continued. I could not convince him to stick with the program once his commitment time was completed.

He moved back to Madison, this time to work at Krystal Hamburgers, and we lost contact for years. It was extremely difficult for me to see him leave the protection of the HMCMHC, but I understood, instinctively, that he must be allowed to live his own life and make his own decisions.

Bernice, my therapist, supported my decision not to spend an excessive amount of energy trying to persuade Bert to do what was obviously against his will. I resigned myself to the reality that there is only so much one can do in our society, even for one who is obviously very ill, if the affected person was not willing to make a commitment of their own.

I understand, though, that Bert was making a commitment of sorts. He had committed himself to trying to live a life independent of the aid that was available to him, in order to become completely self-reliant, and to deny the reality of having mental illness.

While I could respect the strength of will and courage that sort of commitment must take, I could not commit myself to continually trying to dissuade him from pursuing this course. I had to consider my own ability to handle mental strain, which was very much in doubt at that relatively early stage of my recovery.

I remembered the advice of the elderly Southern Belle, who had lived for years on the streets of the Big Apple before returning to Alabama. It was she who had befriended me immediately after I moved into the apartment program from the hospital.

She said, "People are going to do what they're going to do, and I'm flat going to let them."

She repeated this phrase so often that it imprinted in my mind. I could not say whether this was the perfect philosophy or not, but I could certainly see that in those circumstances, it was the only viable option, for me and for everyone counting on me to make the best decisions I could.

My grandmother certainly understood my decision. She applauded the efforts I made to try to help Bert steer himself in the right direction. Unfortunately, Bert had his own ideas about what he considered the right course for himself that were very different from that of his family or the staff of the mental health center.

One day, while on the job at the office of NAMI, I learned that there was a job posting for a peer-support specialist at the state hospital in Decatur, where both my brother and I had been treated. I had visited with the peer support specialist a few times during my stay at the state hospital and found comfort in doing so.

The peer support specialist is a CMHS also, and acts in a quasi-professional role to give advice and hear complaints of clients. The position was part-time, though I felt positive that it could lead to something full-time if the person in that position proved that they could do a good job. The position sounded like a perfect job for me, as I had played a role in the mental health community for a time, and I eagerly filled out an application.

I was overjoyed when I was told that I had been selected to interview for the position, and looked forward, excitedly, to the opportunity. I traveled to Decatur and went into the lobby of the NARH. I was happy to be there for business purposes, rather than for my personal needs or those of my family. There were many people being interviewed, and I realized then just how competitive these positions really were. People of all ages were waiting in the lobby to be interviewed for the one open position.

I remember one man in particular, John, who was waiting to be interviewed. He was probably in his late forties. He seemed like a nice person and we shared our stories. We both hoped to be selected for the position. We realized that we had experiences that allowed us to relate to others, and had the desire to help other people who were in the same situation.

The interview process went well, I thought. I cannot remember all of the questions that they asked me. All I could do was hope that I had some quality they thought would be beneficial to the people they served.

If there was something that would differentiate me from the throng of applicants, who were all qualified, then I really needed it to shine through at that moment.

I awaited the hiring decision while preparing for a trip to Montgomery for a NAMI conference. Then, one morning, something very out of the ordinary happened, but this time it had nothing at all to do with the horrific imaginings related to my symptoms. During this time I took great pleasure in lying in bed in the morning while listening to the radio. I got "hooked" on the Dave Ramsey show, for some reason. Dave Ramsey is a famous radio guru of personal finance. It seems rather ironic now, considering how meager my income was, that I would spend as much time listening to the teachings of Dave Ramsey as I did, yet most of his doctrine is still a cornerstone of my financial knowledge.

On the particular morning in question, I did not awaken to the sobering voice of Dave Ramsey. Instead, what I heard was the description of airplanes crashing into the Twin Towers, the World Trade Center buildings in New York City. I quickly ran to my television set in order to get a better idea of what was happening. As I stared aghast at the television screen, I saw the second airplane hit second tower and envelop it in a ring of fire.

Like most everybody else, I had no idea what was happening, or why. I tried not to become too overwhelmed by the situation, and I think I managed to do so, for the most part, but with one exception.

NAMI courageously decided to go on with their meeting in Montgomery. It met a short time after the events of 9/11, and I, priding myself on my ability to keep things in perspective and not letting world events unbalance me, decided to go with them.

When I arrived at the conference, though, I found myself attending only the opening session and then skipping the rest of the meetings, hoping that the conference participants wouldn't notice my absence. Instead, I stayed fixated on the television set in my hotel room, trying to learn all of the information I could about what had taken place and who had perpetrated it.

The ruins left by the flying bombs and the stories of the courageous police officers and firefighters who tried to save the lives of those trapped in the buildings held me in thrall.

I have always thirsted to learn about current events, especially those involving my homeland, and I could not pull myself away from the gruesome events and their aftermath.

Despite my hopes, everyone noticed my absence from the conference meetings, and I felt quite embarrassed and guilty about the entire affair. It was, of course, wrong for me to accept the scholarship I received to attend the conference if I wasn't going to make a real effort to attend the meetings.

To make matters worse, one of the people who happened to be attending the conference was someone who was a State Advocate for the Department of Mental Health. Jill Russell was a very important person in the mental health community and someone I held in very high esteem, personally. It was her job as a state advocate to hear the complaints of CMHS, who had access to her office. I felt sure she noticed my conspicuous absence and hoped she would not think less of me for my ungraceful neglect of the proceedings.

Not long after this conference, the announcement came regarding the person selected for the peer support specialist position. I was saddened, though not terribly surprised, to learn that it was not me. Although disappointed by the outcome, I felt honored to have even been considered for the position, and I was grateful to have been allowed to participate in this process. The experience did much to kindle hope that perhaps I could find a position such as this in my future.

The country entered a crisis posture, in a sense, after 9/11, and I felt its repercussions like everyone else in the world. Having lived much of my life facing one crisis or another, it deeply distressed me to see the whole world entering a similar state of crisis.

I visited my grandmother, who was in a state of shock about the events that occurred on 9/11. She had lived through interesting times, such as the Great Depression, World War II, and the Cold War, and was horrified to see the nation attacked in such a dastardly way. The enormous personal tragedies she had experienced did nothing to diminish her sense of incredulousness at the events of September 11, 2001.

Grandmother was crowned Queen of the Windsor House nursing home and made President of the Residents Council while I was beginning my twenty-seventh year.

Grandmother had lived long enough to see the world change in many ways, and to experience more than her fair share of misfortune. She had the ability to carry on, though, in the face of the most daunting adversity. Despite the horrible events of 9/11 and the tragedy surrounding her life and her family, she had a unique ability to weather any storm that came her way.

SETTLING IN

During this time, my position on the Consumer Council at the HMCMHC became far more productive than it had ever occurred to me that it could be. Talk began to circulate among the council members about programs known as Consumer Run Drop-in Centers (CRDC). We knew little about these Drop-In Centers other than what we had picked up at the previous Consumer Conference in Shocco Springs. What we did know about them was that CMHS had worked with the state to organize clubhouses, of a sort, in which they could get together, have meals, and plan their own activities.

This sounded interesting to us, as well as to Vickie Hatcher, the staff member of the HMCMHC who advised us on the Consumer Council. She was well liked and respected by all of the clients of the mental health center, and she encouraged us to investigate a CRDC for ourselves to see if it was something we wanted to start in Huntsville.

This was an unexpected turn of events. In my opinion, most of the Consumer Council meetings up to that point had consisted of socializing and trying to think of different fundraising efforts.

All this suddenly changed when instead of selling doughnuts, we were in a van and heading to Tuscaloosa, the home of my Alma Mater, to visit the CDRC that had been established there. This was certainly different from any other trip I had ever taken to Tuscaloosa, but I found the experience to be quite enlightening.

What we found when we arrived there was a small house nestled in one of the neighborhoods, not far from the university campus. I had partied at such houses many times before when I was in college.

We arrived at the Friendship House, Drop-in Center at a time when there were no consumers there, other than the attractive woman who managed the center, Janet. She looked to be my age or younger, and I had seen her at the Consumer Conference in Shocco Springs, though we had not met.

She showed us around the house and explained the types of services they provided. The consumers would socialize, have meals, and plan various activities, she explained. Janet worked part-time to keep the home operating. I don't know if she did this on an entirely voluntary basis, or if she was paid. In either event, I could see that her work in keeping this facility operating made her eminently more qualified to hold a position such as a peer-support specialist or a state advocate with the Department of Mental Health than someone of my limited experience.

The Consumer Council returned from Tuscaloosa with a better idea of what a CRDC was. Then one day, a few months later while at my volunteer job, I came across a handbill similar to the one I had seen posting the peer-support specialist position, though this one listed criteria for starting a CDRC.

The idea began to twist and turn inside my mind, and I decided to call the Alabama State Department of Consumer Relations, which was a branch of the Alabama State Department of Mental Health. It certified a CRDC to be officially sanctioned by the state, and I asked them for the application packet necessary for requesting certification.

When I told the members of NAMI, Huntsville, what I was contemplating, one woman in particular took an immediate interest in the project. Her name was Mary Reeder, and something about the idea of starting a Consumer Run Drop-in Center captivated her imagination as much, if not more, than it did mine.

She was one of the most active members in NAMI, on a state level, and had been for years. She was very prominent in the community, and as I soon learned, proficient in the organizational skills necessary for such an ambitious project. The first thing we did was to organize another trip to visit a completely different Drop-in Center with the members of the Consumer Council who were interested in working on the project.

We carpooled to Gadsden, Alabama to visit their CRDC, and this time we were surprised to find one where many of the consumers came to socialize. It, like Friendship House in Tuscaloosa, was in a small wooden house, and it was certainly thriving.

There were many people of all cognitive functioning levels there having a potluck supper. They seemed to take particular delight in singing karaoke through a large machine they had. Later on that evening, the Drop-in Center presented a special guest speaker who had made a trip there from the state capitol in Montgomery to address the crowd.

Her name was Anne Sawyer, and she was the Commissioner of the Alabama State Department of Mental Health and Mental Retardation. This meant that she was the leader of the mental health system for the entire state.

There in the living room of the small Drop-in Center house, she gave quite an insightful talk that made a lasting impression. She was a middle-aged black woman, and she pointed out the obvious similarities that she saw between the Civil Rights Movement of African Americans, which had made such a powerful impact on the state and nation, and the movement of CMHS, which was going full steam ahead.

She said that she thought that African Americans as a whole had come a long way, in terms of integrating into the larger society, and had come much further than PLMI had been able to thus far.

She said that African Americans had entered a stage of tolerance in the nineteen sixties and was now in the beginning stage of acceptance, with tolerance and acceptance denoting a lower and higher stage of integration, respectively. She said that PLMI were in the beginning stages of tolerance by society and were working steadily to reach the acceptance stage.

The Commissioner then went around the room and asked everyone for input on ways that services for CMHS could improve. She seemed to take great interest in all of our comments, and said that she was intent on implementing the most common themes into policy. We left the meeting feeling richer, in terms of our understanding of what the Consumer Movement could accomplish, and what a CRDC should be. The spark of inspiration to start a Drop-in Center of our own was fanned by our trip into a steady flame.

Events remained stagnant in all other aspects of my life, and I remained largely dissatisfied. I tried to go out to bars once in a while, but was again startled by the type of reception I got from other people when I told them that I had no employment to speak of and spent my time doing volunteer work. I began to drink again, on occasion. After one such outing, I drove home from a bar feeling completely overwhelmed by my situation and completely unable to change it.

I looked to the sky, and I raised my hands and started to weep bitter tears at the seemingly endless stagnancy of the life I lived. I felt sorely tempted to give up hope at that time, but I fixed my mind and soul upon staying faithful to God, who had helped me overcome so many of the obstacles I had already encountered, including close calls with death, and the potential for homelessness, of me and my grandmother.

My therapist, Bernice, was there for me, though, to help me process all of these feelings of dissatisfaction with my life's circumstances and with my shattered view of myself. She listened to my concerns carefully, corrected me when I was being overly negative about myself, and helped me to paint a more accurate portrait of the way I viewed my self-image.

I continued to work on the Drop-in Center project, since I saw it as an opportunity to make life better for all consumers living in my community. A board of directors was formed, and I became the first president. The board consisted primarily of members of the Consumer Council, as well as a consumer named Brian Berry and his wife Darlene. Darlene had managed a women's outreach ministry for a number of years. Mary Reeder, the NAMI Mommy who took an immediate interest in the project, was part of the board as well. She was very prominent in shaping the views of the board and extremely helpful in showing us how to make our dreams become a reality.

The name we all agreed on for our new Consumer Run Drop-in Center was "Our Place."

The most important role I played in the formation of the Drop-in Center was in putting together the paperwork required by the state to show that we were trying to form a CRDC. This amounted to a grant proposal, since, if we were accepted as an official Drop-in Center, we would be eligible to receive state funds which would augment any other monies we could gather for this purpose. The information I had to gather for this was very specific, and included everything from how our board was organized, to how we would raise the additional resources needed to maintain a Drop-in Center.

I was on speaking terms with the man, Mike Autrey, who

essentially made the decisions about Drop-in Centers, and he was also the head of the Office of Consumer Relations. He consented to come and visit the board we had organized.

We met in the NAMI office of the United Way building, and we assured Mike that we were committed to making the Drop-in Center a reality and would work hand in hand with him to see it through. The immediate concern that many on the board had was that we did not have a building to house a Drop-in Center. Mike told us that we were not going to be able to start off having a fully functioning Drop-in-Center with all its amenities, such as the ones in Birmingham and Mobile.

He said that first, we had to start with whatever building we could find to have our meetings. His words rang true as months passed, and we continued to labor and organize. Mary Reeder called a meeting for all consumers, which we held at the First Baptist Church, since she was a long-time member there. The discussion revolved around the topic of the CRDC.

Mike Autrey was invited to the event, and we were all pleased when Mary Reeder informed us that he planned to attend. I was asked to give an opening speech at the event, which I did, writing fiery words about how consumers could organize events and activities for themselves, and that the Drop-in Center was a perfect vehicle for our desire to do just that.

This was a first speech for me, and I felt that it fell flat somewhat, because I was extremely nervous. In any event, a group of about fifty people came to participate, and we were able to demonstrate to Mike that there was genuine interest within the community for a CRDC. Mike spoke to the group about Drop-in Centers and their purpose, and we all felt hopeful about making our vision become a reality in our community.

I told my grandmother about all these activities. My grandmother was, at this time, the oldest surviving member of the First Baptist Church in Huntsville, the place where the meeting was held. Throughout my childhood and young adulthood, her primary method of participation had been as a regular television viewer of the church services; she no longer enjoyed attending the services in person.

I had chosen membership in a different church as a youth, and I grew up in the Church of Christ. However, we always respected one another's right to believe as we chose.

Mrs. Reeder, as well as a surprising number of the NAMI families, had made their home in the First Baptist Church. I was invited to attend a number of artistic functions that the church hosted for the community by the members there, such as Christmas concerts.

Samantha, who provided so much care for my grandmother on a voluntary basis, was a long-standing member of the largest of the Churches of Christ in town, and Grandmother had started over the last few of years, watching the Church of Christ services on television, as well.

Grandmother had spearheaded a large number of philanthropic efforts when she was younger. The one she spoke of most frequently was her part in founding the Burritt Museum. Located atop the green slopes of Monte Sano Mountain, the Burritt Museum showcased a collection of log cabins from different time periods and a variety of animals typically found on farms, among other interesting attractions. It gave me great comfort to be able to inform her that I was working to promote charitable enterprises, as well.

In the middle months of 2001, we were elated to learn that we were certified as an official CRDC by the Alabama State Department of Mental Health. The organization received start-up money amounting to about four thousand dollars. The first thing we chose to spend part of this money on was in hiring an attorney to help us to write papers to file with the IRS to grant us something known as 501(c)3 status, allowing us to operate as a tax-exempt organization.

This is a necessity for any organization operating to provide philanthropic aid. With the help of Darlene Berry, one of the board members, we were also able to locate a house where we could have meetings for several hours each week. Her women's outreach ministry operated full-time to provide spiritual and physical comfort to women who were experiencing abuse.

The women's outreach ministry was located in a house rented by the ministry, and the organization graciously allowed us to have access to their facilities for fourteen hours each week. We all knew that it was a temporary measure, until we could locate a facility of our own. The net result, though, was that we had a Drop-in Center of our own, and Our Place became the place to be for CMHS in the Rocket City.

During this time, I had to make an appearance in court to file bankruptcy on the student loans I had accrued while studying technical writing at UAH. I had to travel to a special bankruptcy court dealing with my student loans, which were considered different from the other debts that had already been discharged by my personal bankruptcy.

The court was located in Decatur, and I drove around the downtown area, once again, in search of the federal courthouse. This time though, it was the middle of the morning, and the circumstances for my being there were far from the romantic encounters with Lorraine that had brought me downtown previously.

After driving in circles around crowded downtown, I located the federal courthouse and found the courtroom where I was supposed to meet my attorney. The only person in the courtroom when I arrived was a bailiff, with whom I talked at length. I was curious about how one went about becoming a bailiff, as it seemed like an interesting job, in my way of thinking. After about twenty minutes, I saw a man whose case was to be heard in front of the court before mine. He was a PLMI who was roughly twice my age, and had worked as a teacher, as well as a security officer in a number of places.

He was trying to file bankruptcy on some student loans, as well. I watched the interplay between this man's attorney, the federal government's attorney, and the judge, and it reminded me very much of the times I had observed court for study purposes in my previous quest to be a law student.

The judge agreed to reduce some of the amount that the plaintiff owed, and I saw this as a good sign for me. It was not long before my case was heard and I was called to the witness stand. The man presiding over the case was very judicious looking, in his bow tie. I found that it was a very different feeling to participate in a court case involving money than it is to merely witness one.

The judge began to question me, and I described all of my life circumstances in detail, including my bid to become a teacher, which had abruptly ended. The judge decided from this that there was no reason I could not continue my endeavor to become a teacher. I was unable to argue with his logic.

It was somewhat unnerving to describe my circumstances to this audience, which included the two attorneys, a middle-aged woman who was the court clerk, the bailiff, and the judge. It was certainly a different experience than my previous one in bankruptcy court, which had been filled with a throng of people and was adjudicated in approximately two minutes.

The judge ruled that I would have none of the six thousand dollars that I owed forgiven, and encouraged me to either continue my education or to figure out some other way to pay the money I owed.

He said that I'd had over eighty thousand dollars of debt forgiven, from hospital bills, mostly, and that I would continue to have to shoulder the remainder of the financial burden. I accepted his judgment with as much dignity as I could muster and thanked my attorney for bringing my case to the court.

In parting from my attorney, who was speaking collegially to the opposing attorney, I shrugged and told him, "Well, I wished we could have settled."

BREAKING THROUGH

I'm standing in a casino in Las Vegas, Nevada, in a sea of video poker and blackjack machines. I've been punching at one particular blackjack machine all day and have won ten dollars in change. Tomorrow we'll leave this entertainment Mecca on bicycle, to continue our Journey of Hope across the desert highway. While I'm in Las Vegas, I cannot help remembering the only other time I was in this city. When I was twelve and my brother Bert was nineteen, my father paid for us to fly out and visit him and his wife here.

Then, as now, I was relegated to the video machines because of my age. Then, as now, I won ten dollars in change. Just as our last trip to Las Vegas, we all had gone the day before to the big water park called Wet'n Wild. On this trip to Wet'n Wild though, I was a chaperone to a twelve-year-old girl, instead of being a twelve year old, myself.

Part of the Journey of Hope was spending time with children with disabilities from various programs. Now, after several hours of riding waterslides of varying dimensions, I couldn't for the life of me figure out what this girl's disability was. Finally, I just asked her in as tactful a way as I could manage, "What is your disability?"

"I have a mental illness." She said without looking at me. She seemed somewhat embarrassed by this, but eventually looked me in the eyes in a determined manner.

"I see." I said in a non-judgmental tone. I couldn't help thinking that this girl looked no different than any other young teenager I'd encountered. I then thought about how difficult it must be for her to go around with the label of having a disability while giving no outward appearance of a problem.

"Well, are you ready to check out that big slide?" I asked.

"Sure!"

She beamed, seeming glad that I had changed the subject. We then padded in our bare feet across the wet concrete and up the next hill.

Back at the video blackjack machine, I took my ten dollar winnings and headed back to my hotel room. "It's just my luck to be in Vegas and not be twenty-one."

"It's very important that you attend our next meeting, Jim," Mary Reeder told me one day around Christmas of 2001, while we were sitting in the offices of NAMI. "Sure, I'll attend," I replied, thinking that she must want me to witness some kind of Christmas celebration, or that she wanted to make sure we had maximum participation at the meeting. I attended the nighttime meeting and discovered, to my delight, that my NAMI family decided to honor me with the Consumer of the Year Award. I received this award for my contributions to the developing of the concept of Our Place, the Drop-in Center we had poured so much effort into. Mrs. Reeder presented the award in front of a conference room full of people who were part of the NAMI family. Whatever choices I ended up making in life, I made with the knowledge that I had the support of these fine people, who had accepted me with open arms.

In the dawn of 2002, the doubt regarding what direction my life was taking began to twist and tighten around my throat, and the screws of regret began to turn. I had not been in a romantic relationship of any sort for a year and a half.

I began to reflect upon the fact that when I had a low wage job previously, I did have some success with women.

When not involved in NAMI activities, my isolation continued, day after long, dull day. I knew I could make something of a full-time commitment to Our Place, one that could likely lead to part-time employment, whenever the Drop-in Center expanded, and perhaps even to employment with the state's available positions to consumers, such as a peer-support-specialist, or a state advocate.

This, though, seemed like a difficult mountain to climb, since I would be working harder while receiving disability payments than I would have without it, and working at a job. It also occurred to me that there was no guarantee for advancement through this strategy, nor was there even any way to know for sure that our dream for a lasting Drop-in Center would even survive. There were several CRDCs we'd heard of which could not be sustained, fading out of existence.

I resumed my exercise of walking as I began to adjust more to the surrounding neighborhood I lived in. I worked out a walking route, which took me through the impoverished environment that surrounded my immediate area and into an oasis of a neighborhood with small, nicely kept houses. Most of these houses had gardens or holiday decorations in their front yards.

Walking through my neighborhood to the oasis neighborhood was somewhat difficult, since were no sidewalks through most of the area. Up to this time, I thought that sidewalks were a common feature to all residential districts in America. I now understood sidewalks to be the luxury they really are.

As with previous periods during which I exercised regularly, I began to experience waves of euphoria and feelings of inspiration. I began to think that maybe it was not too late for me to come up with some plan for a brighter future.

I began filling out a number of job applications at various places.

And with renewed perspective, I also reformed my thinking about what educational opportunities were available to me.

Derrick, the mental health professional who had worked with me at the Day Treatment program in prior years, told me that there was a newly accredited Master's Degree in Social Work (MSW) program that might be worth investigating at Alabama A&M. So I telephoned the university that held this program. The female secretary I spoke with at the social work department certainly seemed encouraging, informing me that I met the basic requirements to be admitted to the program. She said that I could take the Graduate Record Examination, the test most students took to be admitted to graduate school, after I began the program. I would have to sign up for the program soon, though, in order to participate. If I didn't, I would have to wait until next year in order to apply. I also spoke to an adviser in the Education Department at Alabama A&M about obtaining my teaching certificate. I pondered both of these options for gaining future employment during this time. I decided that if I could not find a job I liked at present, then there was no reason for me not to pave my way for a brighter future.

One job I applied for was as a security officer at a plant that made diesel engines for trucks. The advertisement for the position in the newspaper read that the job paid close to ten dollars an hour, which sounded like a veritable fortune to me. I went to the interview and met with executives of a national security company called Vance. These managers had done security work in high-level positions around the country, and seemed very businesslike in their coat and ties.

The man who interviewed me told me that he had begun as a security officer, but had worked his way up to management.

Unlike any other job I had ever heard of, I was provided three days of training for the job, before knowing if I would actually be hired. There were thirty other people in training and none of us knew if we would be hired. We met in a large conference room inside the plant, where we listened to someone explain all of the nuances of guarding a facility. This training was mandatory in order to be considered for one of eight positions. We were told after the training that two other training sessions, containing an equal number of people, had been conducted in order to fill the same eight jobs.

While the large number of people applying for the small number of positions available did not bode well for my chances of obtaining the job, I was encouraged that I had scored a 98% on the written test following the training course.

I was surprised to discover that a large portion of the applicants did poorly on the test and were very disappointed with their scores. However, a week later, the man who would be the security manager at the plant told me that I would not be hired, since all of the positions had been filled. The manager was a former military man, a Vietnam veteran, and the fact that I had no military experience, he implied, weighed heavily against me. I understood this, but I felt disappointed because I was not a person that could even meet the eligibility requirements for military service due to my mental illness.

After another month of applying for jobs and looking at university programs, Glen Bracken, the manager of Vance, who had given me the disheartening news earlier, gave me a phone call. He spoke to me about working for the security company part-time, as a fill in, over the weekends and when other security officers needed time off. He said that in time, it would turn into a full-time position. I was more than elated by this opportunity and quickly agreed to meet with Glen in person.

He seemed pleased to be able to offer the position, and I was sure he could see the joy in my eyes at having a start with Vance. This was a monumental event, in my view, since I was going to go from living on a little less than six hundred dollars per month to earning what amounted to about twenty-thousand dollars a year, whenever the position became a permanent, full-time job.

I was then asked to go and take a drug test, which turned out to be a hair follicle analysis that tested for drug use within the last six months. I had never taken drugs in any serious way, and at this time, I did not drink alcohol any more often than once every couple of months or so. I was grateful that I now could take the drug test with no concern about passing it.

This scenario reinforced my understanding that street drugs are a dead end. Six months prior to landing my job, I had no idea that such a fortuitous opportunity would present itself to me. If I had sought drugs as an escape, even one time in the six months prior to my drug test, my good fortune at going from poverty to a living wage would have been shattered instantaneously.

I received my new security officer's uniform, which I was happy to see was much more stylish than the one I had worn as a security officer at the mall. The uniform consisted of a grey, polo-style shirt and black slacks. The ten-gallon hat I had worn at the Parkway City Mall was mercifully absent.

There was a different atmosphere here. At this post, I guarded a plant full of machinery, which seemed conspicuously empty of the people I thought would have been required to run a large manufacturing plant. Many days and nights, I saw no one other than the other guards working with me on my shift. The job was incredibly tedious, at times, and often involved me watching black and white view screens filled with nothing but the surrounding perimeter for hours at a time. At other times, I was able to pursue my love of walking for exercise, which was only limited by the fact that I had to wear dress shoes. These were harder on my feet than the black tennis shoes I had always worn at Parkway City.

Most of the other officers on the team at the new job were much older than me, and were, for the most part, veterans of the armed forces. A little fewer than half of the officers were close to my age, and two of them were men who were much younger. Several of the officers were retired from high-level engineering jobs who were working until their retirement plans became available. These men were full of wisdom, and I enjoyed talking with them about current events.

At this time, the war in Iraq loomed on the horizon, and enlisted people thought that our country was definitely going to go to war there. I felt that I had made a decisive move in my personal war against my own poverty and lack of life fulfillment. I told my friends at NAMI of my decision to accept this new job, which meant, sadly, that I would be unable to continue with my volunteer job at the NAMI office.

My friends at NAMI in Huntsville, were saddened that I would no longer be at the office, but they seemed to understand that I had made a decision that I thought would be most beneficial to my future. I continued my work with Our Place, although I had no way of investing as much time in it as I would have liked.

I sat in the office of my therapist, Bernice, where so many of my thoughts had been shared, and I talked to her about my good fortune at landing the job. I told her that I was not thinking about additional school anymore, since I had managed to get hired at a job I was happy with.

She seemed to share my joy at having found a way out of the isolation and despair that had been creeping up on me in ever-increasing increments. I felt very much that I was now taking greater control of my own life. Of the many highs and lows I had experienced up to this time, this seemed like one of my happiest moments.

Unless one has experienced poverty and disillusionment for many years, he or she cannot understand the happiness I experienced at this opportunity, which at once propelled me out of the gloom of unemployment and despair.

I understood very clearly that society at large would not consider this a Horatio Alger moment, in which, by “pluck and grit,” a poor young man made it out of misfortune. But it was for me a very clear sign that I did not have to spend my life in poverty. Nor did I have to forego the self-fulfillment that having steady employment can bring. With this understanding, I sent fervent prayers of thanks to my Creator for smiling upon me with the good fortune I had been provided.

One way I expressed the happiness I felt at my change of fortune was by going out on the town; and as was my custom, I went out by myself, or "by my lonesome," as my grandmother would have put it. It had been many months since I had been out, but the fact that I could now strut about with the new confidence of having a job with a good wage, was all the motivation I needed to see the Huntsville lights with my head held high.

This proved to be a more fateful occasion than I could possibly have hoped for, because this was the night I met a person who was to become a very prominent figure in my life. I cannot remember all of the nightclubs I visited in my reunion with Huntsville's night life, but one nightclub in particular certainly stands out in my memory.

The dance club that I visited had undergone many incarnations over the years, as it had a propensity to fall into new owners' hands on an eerily regular basis. While I cannot possibly recall all of the prior names of this club, what I do remember is what it was called on this particular night in question. It was the Breakfast Club, and it had become a theme bar based on the 1980's, replete with giant Rubik's Cubes, a humungous portrait of Al Pacino from the film *Scarface*, and an array of other nostalgic paraphernalia. While I do not remember the 1980's as being especially conducive to dancing and courtship, the novelty was too great for me to pass up such an opportunity.

The first thing that struck me as I looked around the club's dance floors was the fact that the nightclub was conspicuously devoid of patrons. Despite the lack of people, I soon met one of the few attending, and we introduced ourselves.

The woman, whom I will call Sabrina, was an attractive and personable woman who appeared close to me in age, though her young features belied the fact that she was six years older than me. I explained to her that I had a new job, and was out celebrating the fact; and as it turned out, she had just started work at a new job, herself. Her job was quite a bit more prestigious than mine, since she had recently graduated with a degree in computer science, and she had obtained a job in the aerospace industry.

I was too ecstatic with my new job to see this as a great obstacle, and felt encouraged by the fact that we seemed to get along well and had a great deal to talk about. We socialized for a while, and after the "Breakfast Club" closed, we decided to commemorate our new friendship with breakfast at the International House of Pancakes, where we had coffee and continued to learn more about one another.

As it turned out, we had much more in common than we might have first suspected. We had both graduated from the same high school, good old Huntsville High, although she had graduated with an earlier class. Her mother was an Asian American, who had been born and raised in China, and her father was a white American professor. I had gone to my senior prom with an intelligent and lovely Asian American woman, whose family happened to be good friends with Sabrina's family.

Although we had many differences, we had much in common, including our Huntsville roots, and I was happy that our relationship did not end when I telephoned her shortly after this brief encounter. I felt elated that I seemed to have such good fortune in meeting a person I really liked on my first night out after getting my new job.

I didn't bring up the subject of mental illness, as hard-won experience had taught me to avoid this topic until I knew a person for a very long time. I considered the opportunity of getting to know this vibrant woman as something too important to take what I considered the unacceptable risk of revealing everything about my mental health to her, at least right away.

We began to see each other regularly, although I soon discovered that if our relationship was going to become romantic that it was not going to happen in short time. We went out to lunch and dinner and went on walks for a couple of weeks, and then one day Sabrina asked me if I wanted to attend a party with her. I loved parties, although I hadn't been to one in many years. But I was happy to escort Sabrina anywhere she wanted to go.

We arrived at a one-story house, which I was surprised to discover was located only a couple of blocks away from the townhouse where my grandmother and I had lived for much of our lives. I walked into the party with Sabrina, where a large number of people had gathered. I was surprised to discover that no one at this party was drinking.

While I could not claim to have been invited to scores of parties in the past six years, I did not think I was so out of touch with society that the custom of drinking alcohol of some sort had vanished without me noticing. I shrugged this off, intent on having a good time and determined to make a good impression on Sabrina and her friends.

The people gathered at the party all seemed trendy and intelligent, and I began to join the various clusters of conversation with what vigor I was capable of mustering. After talking for about five minutes, I noticed that one of the people began discussing medication that he took for mental illness.

My surprise of one talking so openly about this private matter was mingled with my perpetual caution about revealing anything about my own mental health status. After talking with several other people, I discovered that many of them seemed to be talking about medications and mental health, as well. I walked outside on the front porch to ponder what was shaping up to be a unique turn of events, and felt a weight outside myself pushing me to sit down onto a front porch swing. I realized with dawning clarity that almost everyone at this party was living with a mental illness of some kind. This meant, of course, that Sabrina most likely had mental illness of her own, as well.

My mind was reeling with all of this new revelation, as Sabrina sat down on the swing next to me, and began talking to me about her own mental illness. This shocking discovery was like being splashed in the face with a bucket of water, and I thought to myself that our meeting must have been fate. I then thought, surely I must be meant to fall in love with this person.

She brought me to this party as her way of revealing to me that she had mental illness, and I thought, "Just wait until she discovers that I, myself, have mental illness too." Holding on to my own secret now seemed like the sheerest folly, and so, with a faint and stammering voice, I told her.

"Sabrina, you know, I have a mental illness of my own. It's schizophrenia."

She then said something that startled me as much as anything else I had witnessed so far.

She said, "I knew you had mental illness before I brought you to this party."

"Really?" I said, "How could you have known that?"

She then said, with a smile on her face, "Do you remember when we ate at the Olive Garden for lunch the other day?"

"Yes."

Sabrina grinned, "You took your keys out of your pocket, and when you did I noticed on your key chain there was a NAMI logo."

"No kidding," I said.

I did not even remember placing such a device on my perpetually filled key ring, but when I pulled out my key chain to examine it, the big blue capital letters, NAMI, on a white plastic rectangle, were there in plain view.

Sabrina's powers of observation were far superior to mine, in many respects, and she had used them to create a day to be remembered in the lifetime of a person who has been witness to many strange and wondrous events.

NORMAL ALABAMA

I spent one more glorious week dating Sabrina, now armed with the knowledge that we both were living with mental illness. What I learned of Sabrina was that she had an inspirational story. She had attended an Ivy League college and had eventually gone on to become accepted to medical school.

While at medical school, she had been diagnosed with schizophrenia, and had gone back home to live with her parents, just as I had following my own diagnosis. After allowing time to become accustomed to her new situation, she then attended UAH for four years to earn a new bachelor's degree in computer science. She had now come to the end of this difficult and triumphant path, and had been hired in a technical position. Though it took time and struggles, she learned to cope with mental illness, and to renew her professional life.

I was moved by her inspirational story, since up to this time I had never met any person with the type of mental illness we had who had managed such a feat. We went on walks through the wooded Monte Sano Mountain, which I had been to so many times during my youth. We both enjoyed walking for our exercise, and each other's company. During these walks, we discussed plans I had for my future. I had told her of my original intention of becoming a lawyer, and explained to her that I had pursued the teaching profession, once upon a time, as well.

I let her know, also, that I sometimes thought about entering the social work profession, to become a psychotherapist. For now though, I was interested only in basking in the glory of my new security job. We hit many yard sales, where she enjoyed looking at the endless array of items, which she loved to collect. On one such occasion, we went to a house in an up-scale neighborhood where a woman Sabrina had known from high school was clearing out the family home of her parents, who had recently passed away.

To my surprise, the woman remembered my brother, Bert, who had lived in the neighborhood for a short time as a child. I had no knowledge of the neighborhood or that my family had once lived in a house there.

It reminded me once again that Bert had an early childhood very different from my own. He had lived a life with my mother and father when times were good for them, when they had been a cohesive family unit living in a "ritzy" neighborhood. His childhood was very different from the disjointed bouncing around of my own early years. After my parents' divorce, Bert went from a traditional nuclear family unit, straight into foster homes and poverty.

While driving away from this yard sale, I felt compelled to tell Sabrina everything I had been through involving my brother, Bert. She was from a tightly knit family unit, as is the case with most families with Asian roots, and she did not interpret my relationship with my brother in the same way I did. Despite all of my explanations, she could not fathom the idea that Bert and I would not be on speaking terms.

A few days later, Sabrina consented to go with me to visit my grandmother at Windsor house, and I was happy that they could get to know one another, as I now considered Sabrina an important part of my life.

One situation she wanted remedied, to which I eagerly agreed, was for me to quit smoking cigarettes. I had been addicted to nicotine for over four years, by that time, and I knew it was a terrible idea for me to continue smoking. I had been a smoker ever since I had been a patient at the state hospital, and my jobs in security, which entailed constant exercise, had not curbed my craving for cigarettes in the slightest.

I stopped smoking, cold turkey, because I valued my relationship with Sabrina more than I did my love affair with nicotine. One night on her couch, I trembled and shook visibly, feeling the chills of nicotine withdrawal, which I felt had to be as bad as withdrawal from any other drug. My long-term goal to stop smoking coincided with my long-term goal of continuing my relationship with Sabrina. She seemed pleased by my gesture and encouraged me to maintain abstinence from smoking.

Despite my best efforts, our romantic relationship was to be short-lived. Sabrina said that she was not interested in pursuing the course that

I thought inevitable. Being persistent, I continued to telephone Sabrina to plead my case, but I was met with refusal.

One thing I discovered in all of this, was that despite the fact that Sabrina was unwilling to engage in a romantic relationship, she continued to remain a good friend. I continued to telephone her in an effort to kindle a romantic relationship, and instead of cutting me out of her life completely, she continued to not only hear my pleas, but also to talk to me for about as much time as I cared to. We talked on the telephone for at least two hours every day. We still spent time together, going places, though not as much as we did before, and although my disappointment at the turn of events was palpable, it was tempered with an equal measure of joy that I had a new friend.

My ability to remain nicotine-free proved to be inadequate. I managed to remain free of cigarettes for another couple of weeks after Sabrina's decision not to date me until something peculiar happened.

One day while driving, I could have sworn I saw Bert, or someone who looked very much like him, walking across the street, maybe fifty feet in front of my car. Something about this experience triggered an instantaneous and irresistible desire for me to stop at the gas station only a block away and buy a pack of cigarettes, which I immediately began lighting as if I had never quit. I told Sabrina about my inability to stop smoking the next day. She was disappointed, but she remained my friend.

I was introduced to Sabrina's network of friends, who tended to be highly intellectual, some of whom had mental illness they were living with, and some of whom did not. While I was out of touch with socialization of any sort with people my own age, I certainly had not tended to spend time socializing with individuals of the intellectual persuasion, even before I was diagnosed with my mental illness. It was refreshing to spend time with these people, as I found acceptance from them that I had never really received from most fraternity and sorority members I had mingled with in my college days.

I remember going to the movie theater with this group to see the film version of Oscar Wilde's play, *The Importance of Being Earnest*. I had read the play years before, and I did not laugh as much as the other people in the movie theater, as I already knew much of what would happen. However, I now understood what it was like to interact with the "art house crowd," and discovered that I enjoyed this interaction much more than I did interacting with people of different tastes. Mainly though, I interacted with Sabrina, and we continued to learn more of each other's life stories.

The benefit of my finding someone I both related to and admired was immeasurable. Although I continued to begrudge the lack of romantic love, the limbo of isolation that had enveloped my life began to recede.

My life was looking up in a number of ways as I continued down a new path. I remember walking around the plant where I worked, through the maze of incomprehensible machinery in the middle of the night's blackened glow. I thought that perhaps I should write a letter to my stepfather, since I had not contacted him in about a year and a half.

I thought, "Yes, I should write him and let him know I decided to settle on the simple life that he had suggested to me on the front steps of NARH." He had asked me to describe the good points of working at the Holiday Inn and had suggested that it was a good job for me. I wanted to let him know that I had even met friends who were intellectual, like him. I thought long and hard about sending him this letter, but I never wrote it.

I was also working with men who were a decade or so younger than my stepfather, who were retired engineers.

One of them, whom I will call Gary, confided in me that it broke his heart that I and the other young men in the job, all of whom he thought had great potential, were choosing to stay in that job instead of pursuing some professional occupation.

I accepted his opinion, but felt that he did not understand my struggle, especially in light of the fact that I had a serious mental illness. I was not willing to explain it to him. I was quite surprised by his frank and emotional words, though, especially since we had enjoyed only a working friendship. His words echoed Sabrina's, who thought that I had the potential to pursue the law degree I had originally intended, or a degree toward some other profession. I continued to see primarily the hills and mountains I had already traversed, though, and was reluctant to allow my mind to wander toward the new horizons of an unknown profession.

While all of this was taking place, I continued seeing my therapist,

Bernice, and discussing the events taking place in my life. I told her that I had decided to settle on this new life, working for a wage that I enjoyed very much, especially since there were new changes in Medicare that allowed me to keep my health insurance for a longer time.

She listened patiently as we continued our sessions. Sometimes I mentioned the possibility of pursuing a MSW degree, which she had earned to become a therapist. This was only an idea I "bounced off of her," though. I continued to be content with my new situation, and I was not willing to risk it in any way.

Whenever I did mention this idea though, she had a way of teasing it out to the point that I could see it more clearly, by her asking me specific questions. After our sessions, I began seeing the idea as more and more of a real possibility, and was encouraged that she didn't seem to see any reason why I could not pursue this goal.

My sense of self-esteem remained terribly low, and she had a way of bolstering my vision of self so that I did not feel as utterly devoid of confidence in pursuing such a profession. I suppose that having good therapists, in one sense, was a deterrent to me having a goal of entering their ranks. I didn't know how I could ever live up to their amazing example. They had saved my life and helped me to feel like a worthwhile person. Did I have the ability to help other people in the same way?

I pondered this idea more and more often, and soon found that I was struggling with whether or not to pursue it. In 2001, this new job was a greater opportunity than I'd had in a long time, and I was now twenty-seven years old. My failure to successfully further my education in 1999 remained fresh in my mind. I knew for certain that it would be unwise for me to try to work full-time and pursue a graduate degree, since there would certainly be conflict between work and school hours. As things stood, I was called randomly to work for Vance International, at any hour of the day. I counterbalanced those tangible doubts with the clear faith in me exhibited by my therapist and co-workers.

I telephoned the Social Work Department at Alabama A&M the way I had one year before to ask them about applying to the program. Like the last time, they said that I would have to apply soon in order to be accepted in the program for the year.

I now faced one of the most agonizing decisions of my life. I sat in

Bernice's office holding my head in my hands, thinking about what the best decision for me would be, understanding, instinctively, that she could not tell me what I should do, but only help to guide my own decision-making process.

I discussed these options with my grandmother, who was equally reluctant to tell me specifically what I should do. Not even Sabrina would tell me whether I should choose social work over some other pursuit.

One aspect to security work that I have alluded to is that guards often have a great amount of time to ponder the course their life will take. The physical exercise of much walking, which is certainly a key component of security work, helps create moments of euphoric clarity in which one can really get in touch with the higher power as well as his own dreams. It was during one such moment of clarity and vision when I realized that I had a higher calling. This higher calling was to become a psychotherapist and a social worker. I said to myself, "I think that this is what God really wants me to do."

It was not exactly like Paul, traveling on the road to Damascus, where he was convinced by God to set his life on a new course. It was much more subtle than that. I realized that everything in my life had seemed to prepare me for this particular path. My road to Damascus had occurred on the highways and byways where I had blistered my feet straining to understand God's Voice, although it had taken me six years to understand where it led. Paul did not require two roads to Damascus, and Jonah did not need to be swallowed by a great fish more than once. These men were much older than I was when they chose to understand their higher calling, which was for them to use the talents they discovered they had in their attempt to make the world a better place.

I could spend my time and energy honing my talents to help people overcome the same obstacles I'd had to contend with. I realized that it was worth me risking yet another failed attempt at success in order to make this happen. This dream was not about my own ambition for personal gain, but instead about how I could help other people. I realized, though, it was an opportunity for personal growth, as I worked to make the world a better pace for PLMI and their families.

My confidence in myself was still at a rather low point, despite the encouragement and friendship that I had from so many fine people in my life. My faith in this new endeavor was enormous, though. I knew it was a path that I had to pursue, despite any self-doubt. I would be faithful to my dream and trust in God to deliver me to the higher plane in which I would become an effective servant to others.

I handed in my resignation letter, which weighed heavily in my hand, to my boss Glen, and explained to him my decision to pursue my dream. Perhaps he had suspected I would do this from the moment he hired me, and perhaps he did not. What is certain, though, is that the confidence he displayed in hiring me did a great deal in terms of helping to propel my life on to a new course.

The plant for which our company supplied guards was located right next to the Huntsville International Airport, and we had occasion to see airplanes taking off and landing on a regular basis. I had now become, figuratively speaking, one of the large jets that was departing the airport to fly into parts unknown, and like those airliners I would be providing passage to as many souls as I could carry to destinations of recovery from serious mental illness.

I was now breaking new ground in personal growth and embarking on a journey to aid others on their own paths to recovery. I had faith in God to aid me in this quest, and I knew without question that I would do nothing to let myself down, nor the people who had faith in me. I would use every ounce of my energy and commitment to make my dream to help other PLMI a reality by becoming a part of a profession perfectly designed to do just that.

I had learned many life lessons, and had experienced enough of the world to realize that I could use my knowledge of recovery to benefit others. I was fortunate enough to have been given the wisdom to realize my own potential to make my life one of greater purpose than it had ever been. It had been two and a half years since I had given up my pursuit of becoming a teacher and made the decision to live on disability insurance. The sadness and feelings of desperation I experienced during that period of time would never be entirely forgotten.

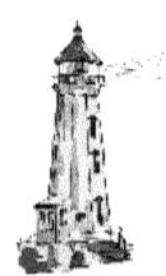

LIFE LESSONS

In the fall of 2002, I attended the orientation session for my new classes, with an eager heart and a curious mind. The creed of Alabama A&M is "Service is Sovereignty," and I could tell at once that I was now in the right place at the right time. A&M is located in a northern suburb of Huntsville, in an area called Normal, Alabama. It is a proud member of the Historically Black Colleges and Universities located throughout the nation, and it is one of the oldest Universities in the state. The demeanor of the professors and the information they provided at the orientation session bolstered my resolve to pursue my MSW, and served to strengthen my feeling that I had finally found my niche.

One thing that was likely apparent to the people around me was my sense of thankfulness that I had the opportunity to be a part of this program. I was, in effect, bound to my geographical location, because I didn't intend to move very far away from my grandmother. Up until about five years earlier, the only school that had a MSW program was the UA.

I was impressed immediately by the educators, who started the MSW program at Alabama A&M. They assured me that creating the MSW program was no simple matter. The program had only been accredited, which is a very important factor for social work education, for a few years. Everyone who graduated before that time was able to be grandfathered in for accreditation. I was also impressed by my new professors' ability to explain the details of the MSW program and the licensure process in a straightforward way.

I began my courses in earnest, and soon realized that I was going to have an enormous amount of work to do. I was expected to write a seemingly endless number of papers. This was also the case for my failed attempt at technical writing school; although I realized that unlike technical writing, in social work I had an infinite number of subjects to write about.

Since I had no prior experience in social work, I spent my first two semesters learning about my major, such as what it entailed, and some of the basics of its practice. Unlike many of the other students who had no idea of what type of work they wished to do once they graduated, I knew without question: I wanted to be a mental health counselor.

I had to wait until my second year, however, to begin really learning the specifics of mental health social work, and how to treat different mental illnesses with specific approaches to therapy.

The makeup of the faculty, as well as the majority of students, were female. About half of them were black, and the other half white. There were also students from other countries, who brought their own unique perspectives to social work study. I was surprised to see that I was not the oldest student there, and was happy to see that there were students of all ages. It was clear that many of the students there were similar to me in the sense that they did not have a straight path to their choice of social work as a profession, but had come to this conclusion over time, through winding routes.

I was likely considered somewhat eccentric by many people there because of my lack of socialization, and my somewhat different set of experiences and life views. It was clear at first though, to teachers as well as students, that my knowledge base on most of the issues discussed was extensive. I poured myself into my studies and was pleased that I was rewarded with high marks as a result.

One experience of note occurred during my first semester in the form of my participation in an undergraduate class. I had never taken a biology course in my undergraduate studies, and now had to do so in order to meet the requirements of the master's degree. I attended the class in an auditorium and was somewhat surprised to discover that I was the only white person in the room, and certainly one of the oldest students there. The black woman who taught the course accepted me graciously, as did the young students who surrounded me. It did not take me long to realize that I was fortunate, indeed, to be able to have such an experience, and felt that other white students in the United States would benefit from a similar one.

I had a sense of being a minority in a sea of people different from me. Just walking around the campus, surrounded by people of different ethnicities created a paradigm shift that I was quick to notice, and helped me to gain a better understanding of what it must be like for black people or other members of racial minorities each day throughout their lives. As soon as I left the campus, I was back in a world where most people tended to look similar to me, and I realized that this campus must feel as something of an oasis to people of color.

I was a member of a minority myself, as a PLMI, though this was not apparent to the observer, and I tended not to announce having a mental illness. I broke my propensity toward silence about my illness, though, within a couple of weeks after beginning my new courses.

One professor in particular seemed to conduct herself in an especially understanding way. She asked us to write a paper about ourselves, and I took the opportunity to describe what it was like to have a mental illness. Later, she asked me to come to her office and spoke to me about what I wrote in the paper. Professor Harris was in her early forties, with a tall, attractive frame and a very disarming personality.

"So, you are on all of your medications, right?" she asked.

"Yes, I am," I said.

"So you've already been through all of that, huh?" she questioned with a smile.

"Yes, that's right," I laughed.

I then told her my whole story. I was relieved to be describing my circumstances to this woman and to feel her acceptance pour into me.

Within the month, the annual Alabama Mississippi Social Work Conference was to take place in Tuscaloosa, and I was one of the students who chose to attend. I certainly did not have the funds to pay for a hotel room, but I felt that I had a way around this by merely spending one night in my old fraternity house, located about two blocks away from where the conference took place. It had been about five years since I had even visited the old fraternity house, and about six years since I had spent the night there—and that was when I was experiencing a psychotic break with reality. Since then, I had experienced recurring dreams in which I woke up in my old fraternity house, as if I had never experienced mental illness and was resuming my college attendance.

When I got to Tuscaloosa, the men at the fraternity house welcomed me as an alumnus and were very hospitable. I experienced the most palpable feeling of déjà vu as I ate dinner with these young men in the big dining hall on the immense wooden tables and socialized with them.

Walking around the old parlor—which had been remodeled and looked better than ever—evoked feelings of nostalgia as I looked at the hardwood floors and old decor.

When I explained to these youthful fraternity brothers that I was there to attend a social work conference, I could tell by their reactions that the entire notion of this seemed alien. One of them loaned me his room for the night, so that I might have a place to lay my head. The feeling of surrealism at sleeping on a bed in my old fraternity house washed over me like a nostalgic wave. I drifted off to sleep with great expectations for the next day.

I attended the Alabama Mississippi Social Work Conference happy to meet with the people fellow attendees, and thankful that this new chapter of my life was well underway. I remember one meeting at the conference in particular, in which a knowledgeable, charismatic black man conducted. He offered a bag of chips to everyone and I eagerly raised my hand. I reached inside the bag and when I pulled it out, I was excited to discover I had grabbed several dollars. The speaker had done this to illustrate the lesson that opportunities occur to people who are willing to receive them.

Although I felt fortunate to have the financial advantages that I did during this time, including my disability payments and my housing subsidy, I continued to struggle financially. The old adage about starving students certainly held true for me; I would go from times of having plenty of money to those where I had to choose between eating and smoking cigarettes. I had not really experienced this level of poverty since I had been a child in the slums of Oregon, and was rather amazed that many of the other students, who did not even have the same economic advantages that I now had, were managing to survive during their studies.

I started socializing with people at a bar. I was with a former high school classmate, who was an investment banker, along with some of his friends. They didn't seem to understand my decision to pursue social work. I did my best to talk to them about topics of similar interest and to keep up with them in their heavy drinking. Our association abruptly ended though one night, when I drank so much that a certain song on the radio began to make me visibly weep. Later that night, after almost getting into a fight with someone for no reason at all, I drank one drink too many, and something in my mind gave way to the point at which I began to lose all focus of the world around me.

This was a very frightening experience, and I realized for the first time since I had resumed drinking socially that I was quite limited in the amount I could drink.

The second semester of school began, and I spent the first two weeks trying to get my mind back in focus, which, thankfully, I eventually did before any of my assigned work was due.

I didn't return to the bar that my new friends frequented during that "cooling off" period, but when I finally did return, I found that my abrupt absence, perhaps combined with my behavior on my bender, resulted in a cool reception by my newly acquired companions. I felt even more like an oddball in their presence because I knew for certain I could not drink nearly as much as they could. After that, I would drink socially on occasion; however, I always did so with the knowledge that alcohol was definitely not good for my psychological condition. Over time I tended to drink increasingly less, as thoughts about my mind buckling under the pressure of alcohol were ever-present in my mind.

These young business professionals were certainly not the only people who spent time at this bar. People who worked in all manner of occupations spent time there. I found that many of them did not respect my chosen profession either. One waitress in particular whom I tried to make time with identified social work with people who were involved with child custody cases, which is certainly one important aspect of what social workers do.

While I had no particular ambition to be involved in that type of social service, I was identified with those people, nonetheless. I discovered that I was disliked by some who considered social workers to be "baby snatchers." I soon decided that hanging out at the bar was really not good for me. Instead, I decided to spend more time alone, focused on my studies. Any desire to meet and socialize with people in nightclubs for any length of time never returned. With every passing year, I found myself feeling more alienated in that environment.

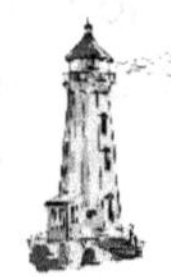

NEW BEGINNINGS

After launching back into studies for the second semester at A&M, I received a telephone call from my friend Sabrina. She said that she had someone with whom she wanted to arrange a date for me. I readily agreed to the proposal. I was very appreciative of Sabrina's thoughtfulness, especially since I had not been in a serious relationship with a woman in about three years.

The woman I went on the date with was a full-figured brunette in her late twenties, whom I will call Roxanne. She was from the Ukraine, and had lived in the United States for about eight years with a couple from her church. We had an instant rapport, and I was happy to find myself in a new romantic relationship, at last. Neither Sabrina nor I told her about my mental illness, and I continued my habit of waiting until I thought the time was right to let her know everything about my mental health status.

I learned that she was very involved in her church, which was a conservative branch of Presbyterian. Her church was responsible, through their mission work, for Roxanne's presence in this country. Roxanne had converted to Christianity in her native Ukraine, and then moved to the United States where she lived with her foster family and attended college. She had earned her degree in International Studies from the UAH and was now working in customer service at a large bank, as well as working at a couple of other part-time jobs. Her religious life was very important to her, and since I considered myself a very spiritual person, I was no stranger to attending church.

I soon began attending church services with her. As our relationship progressed, I even became a member of the church, though my views tended to be a bit more liberal than the official church dogma. Roxanne was more conservative than me in many of her life views, but we were able to live with these differences for the sake of our relationship.

My second semester of graduate school passed by quickly, as I prepared to begin the direct practice of social work skills. This required working for three semesters at internships, known as field practicum. The woman who was in charge of the field practicum program was a middle-aged black woman, named Professor Mclynn, who also happened to be one of the most personable people I had yet to meet. She told me that she wanted me to work at the Morgan County DHR, located in Decatur, as a prelude to field practicum at a mental health facility.

DHR for each county was responsible for working for its citizens with child custody cases, as well as other matters. I agreed with my advisor that it would be an educational experience for me to learn more about other areas covered by social work besides mental health. My first memories as a child had been of foster homes and the social worker who was involved in my case. Mrs. Butler, whose white hair matched the white of the tiny jeep she would drive me around in as she helped decide my fate through my childhood years, was a pivotal figure in my recollection. She made her presence known at key points throughout my childhood when she would mediate the decisions made by myself and my family.

I believed also that this profession was being demonized unnecessarily, and I wanted to try to learn more about why. My barroom acquaintanceships, which had ended up with me feeling ostracized because of my chosen field of study, had piqued my curiosity about this as much as anything else.

I remembered my grandmother and stepfather's fears of the mental health system, which certainly had in my own experience proven to be false. I also recalled my grandmother's dissatisfaction with the DHR. She had been greatly displeased with their decision to remove my brother and myself from my mother's custody and to send us to foster care. My grandmother's level of frustration about the situation was increased by the fact that DHR would not allow her to take over the custody of her own grandchildren, herself.

I was eager to get started in my work for the DHR in Morgan County, happy to be going to the River City of Decatur for yet another reason that didn't involve me being hospitalized.

My relationship with Roxanne progressed. However, I remained unwilling to inform her of my diagnosis with schizophrenia. She did not share my interest in social work, but she was supportive of me pursing my field of study.

One feature of my new responsibilities was that I now had a good reason to purchase a cellular phone. I had lived well below the poverty line for the majority of my adult life. The only time I had even for an instant considered purchasing a cell phone had been in the middle of a psychotic break in 1998, when I had abruptly left my workstation at the Holiday Inn front desk to go traipsing around the nearby mall.

It was now 2003, five years later, and I had not considered trying to buy a cell phone since then. In fact I became quite embarrassed whenever I was even around a cell phone because I had no idea of even how to dial a call on one of those devices.

It seemed to me that practically everyone I encountered had a cellular phone, and in some cases, even young adolescents and children seemed to be chatting on them. It was with pride, then, that I walked into the Verizon store and was happy to discover that I was eligible to purchase my first cell phone. My delight was not only over possessing a new gadget, but also because I now had a reason for needing a cell phone, since the work I would be doing would be improved if I had access to greater means of communication.

I wanted to make a good impression on my new colleagues, and I believed that having a cell phone would allow me to do a better job. I examined the features of the phone, all of which were foreign to me; but now that I owned one, and had a moment to examine my phone closely, I caught on to how it operated.

My field practicum at the Morgan County DHR took place in the summer, and I worked for forty hours a week there and took two classes at night.

This was definitely a departure from the hours of free time I had on my hands in the period when I did only volunteer work. Before I could begin my work with this agency, though, I had to be interviewed.

The interview went well, other than the initial difficulty I had in locating the agency. The woman who interviewed me was tall and thin with translucent-looking blond hair. The years of service she had provided to families could be seen on her expression, which seemed scoured of concerns for anything other than doing her job. One of the first questions she asked was whether I wanted to work for the Child and Family branch of the agency or at the Adult Services department. I instantly answered that I would rather work for the Adult Services branch of the agency, which worked to protect the rights and health of adult citizens from abuse and neglect.

My decision was based, in part, on the fact that I was responsible for the care of an elderly person, my grandmother, and I felt more inspired to pursue this course than to be involved in the affairs of parents and children. This was especially the reason, because my ultimate goal was to get a position working with adults with serious mental illness. The woman who interviewed me respected my decision; although, she said she was disappointed by it. "There are just not enough people who want to do this type of work with children and their families," she said. "You can have a position working in Adult Services, then." She sighed.

Unlike my decision to inform the professors at my school of my mental illness, I did not feel a similar compulsion to inform the Department of Human Resources of this fact. I felt that this might create awkwardness, even if only in my own mind, and I did not want to take any chances on limiting employment opportunities.

The people at DHR accepted me, and I appreciated the atmosphere there and was thankful to even have my own office, which included a computer and a telephone. As a student intern, I did not have anywhere near the amount of responsibility and workload of the other staff, and it did not take me long to recognize that the staff felt a great deal of stress and burden regarding the important work and decisions they had to make daily.

The years of stifling despair that had plagued me were now counterbalanced with a wave of hope for the possibility of a successful future. I made the decision to quit smoking at that time, and started chewing nicotine gum as a substitute.

My work duties began with visiting elderly people, or adults with other disabilities, who had great difficulty in caring for themselves. I did everything from grocery shopping for a woman who was in sole charge of a brother who was entirely disabled; to helping a man obtain an air conditioner; to visiting people in a nursing home, who had no one else to visit them. I walked through low-income project areas some of the time, much the same way I had when I worked for the Census Bureau in 2000.

It dawned on me that there was a vast underbelly of society that was in dire need, and had problems with disability and poverty. I was becoming someone who was on both the receiving and giving end of the resources in place to assist them.

It occurred to me often that it was not that long ago when I was sitting in the lobby of Madison County in Huntsville, waiting for my own appointment to receive food stamps.

When I saw people in the lobby at DHR in Decatur who were waiting to talk about food stamps or some other concern, I did not feel like a person outside their social sphere. I had no problem relating to them in terms of the vexing toll that poverty can have on the human psyche.

I realized that most of society knew nothing of the suffering and hardships that their less fortunate brothers and sisters experienced on a daily basis. Many of them would never know about this underworld of people in need unless, like me, they found the circumstances of their lives interrupted by some life-altering event.

My work at DHR also included, to my great surprise, assistance to the people who worked for the Child and Family branch of the agency. Women who worked for this service walked into homes that might be dangerous, and they felt much more comfortable going into the unknown with a large man at their side.

I made a point to stay uninvolved in the interviews that took place in these households, since I knew my experience in this area was limited. I was pleased to have a bird's eye view of these proceedings and to learn more about social work and child welfare in general.

What I learned was that it had become extremely difficult to remove a child from the custody of a parent in Alabama. Even if custody is removed, DHR looks for people like grandparents or other relatives to care for the child first. If I had been in the DHR system of 2003 as a child, I would have been allowed to live with my grandmother, and my first memories would not have been of foster parents.

After dating for eight months, I felt comfortable enough with our relationship to tell Roxanne about my mental illness. We were outside of a Mexican Restaurant where we had just dined, and I broke the news to her in the gentlest way I knew how.

She did not take the revelation well, and to my horror, she burst into tears upon hearing the facts. Our relationship ended in very short order. After about two weeks, she telephoned and our relationship resumed for a month or so. But in the end, the fact that I had a serious mental illness was simply too much for her to handle.

Doubtlessly, our relationship was also tenuous because I was still a student, despite the fact that I was doing unpaid work and continued to have little idea whether I would find a position, or how much it would pay, whenever I did find one. The school assured me I would not have difficulty finding employment, and that the salary would be quite a lot more than I expected it to be. My grandmother had taught me to "never count your chickens before they hatch," and I remained skeptical to a degree on what kind of career opportunity would surface.

After a memorable summer, I ended my service with the Morgan County DHR, thankful for the opportunity to work and learn with the people there and with the people I had served. After a year of learning the basics of social work intervention, I looked forward to starting the first semester of my second year at A&M, where I began to learn the "nuts and bolts" of providing social work in a mental health setting.

My next internship took place at the mental health center in Decatur. My journey into achieving my dream of learning to become a psychotherapist was now fully underway and I looked forward to learning everything I could in my quest to make this dream become a reality.

GRADUATION

I drove to Decatur once again to be interviewed for a field practicum at the mental health center, which served Morgan County. The Decatur Morgan Counseling Center (DMCC), was nestled between the Wallace Center, a vast compound that was residence for hundreds of people with mental retardation, and NARH, with which I had become intimately acquainted. In many ways, Decatur seemed to be a kind of Mecca for mental health services of all kinds, and I felt that it was the right place for me to be.

A friendly woman named Gloria conducted the interview. She was the Clinical Director of the Mental Health Center of North Central Alabama (MHCNCA), the organization that oversaw DMCC. This meant that she was in charge of the people who provided direct care for the clients for three counties, as the MHCNCA was responsible for providing services in Morgan, Limestone, and Lawrence Counties.

She asked questions about my work background and described the types of services the center offered. She then began showing me around the center, including the area where I would be working, known as Day Treatment. She said she was particularly proud of the area and that no expense was spared in its operation. I had been a client in the Day Treatment program in Madison County for a time, years earlier, and was certainly familiar with the services offered, but I didn't feel compelled to explain this to her at that time. I chose instead to keep the knowledge of having a mental illness to myself.

I was backed by this decision by my own therapist, Bernice, who compared having mental illness with having a heart condition or any other physical illness. One would certainly feel no obligation to inform one's prospective employer of a physical condition of this kind, unless the condition would adversely affect performance on the job.

I freely acknowledge that romantic relationships are a much different matter, and different people will have different ideas about what information should be disclosed and when; but in the area of employment there is no moral ambiguity in my mind, and certainly none under the law.

I was soon introduced to the woman who coordinated the Day Treatment program at the DMCC, and who would be my boss. Her name was Trish, and we developed an almost instant rapport. I was also introduced to her boss, Mike, the program director for the DMCC. He was a wise and amiable man, nearing retirement.

I then began the actual work of my internship and began meeting the clients I would be working with. I was immensely excited by the prospect of being able to work on their behalf, and was pleased to find that I had an almost instant connection with them.

I thought, "This is great! I'll have this instant rapport with all of the clients because of our shared experiences of symptoms and overwhelming despair, but no one will realize exactly why."

I thought that this hidden advantage could be a decisive factor in me being viewed as a particularly effective mental health worker. I did not reveal directly to the clients that I had a mental illness, but was able to converse at length on practically any issue they brought to my attention.

The therapist acts as an agent for change within the client, and the mental health status of the therapist is not important, in and of itself, except to the extent that it helps him or her to empathize with what the client is experiencing.

Day Treatment is a program that clients can attend four hours a day from two to five days a week in order to receive group and individual therapy. Here, clients also attend classes on coping with symptoms of their mental illness and receive rehabilitative training in a variety of areas. Typically, the clients who attend Day Treatment are considered to be at high risk for relapse from their illness. As a result, they were hospitalized repeatedly. They were on various levels, in terms of cognitive functioning, but for the most part, those who participated in Day Treatment for long periods were the ones that faced extreme difficulty in terms of managing the symptoms of their mental illnesses from day to day.

I soon realized that the Day Treatment Program was the crown jewel of the entire organization. There was no shortage of resources for the clients and there was a wide array of services, as well as the opportunity to participate in exciting activities. Friday was fun day, when the clients could get away from the day-to-day tedium of attending therapy groups. On most Fridays, the client's engaged in fun activities such as playing bingo or singing karaoke, and the staff worked to prepare a big meal for them. On other Fridays the clients went on trips to parks, museums, ate out, or went bowling. Day Treatment was a window for these clients, normally stranded by lack of transportation and financial resources, to the outside world, to save them from the desolation of their own four walls.

Two days a week, a volunteer worked in the program to teach the clients who needed to earn the equivalent to a high school diploma, known as the G.E.D. It delighted me tremendously to see these clients, some who would likely never be able to earn a G.E.D., work to improve their reading and math skills. I was also inspired, because the person who taught the class was a woman struggling with a serious mental illness of her own. She had once worked as a special education teacher in a public school.

One of the greatest benefits of Day Treatment was the interaction that took place between the clients. It was quite a wonderful sight to see clients, who without Day Treatment were otherwise isolated, engaging in social activities with one another. They encouraged each other, and demonstrated kindness to one another in a variety of small ways.

One downside to this situation was that eighty percent of the people I was now surrounded by smoked cigarettes and this contributed mightily to my all too hasty decision to pick up cigarette smoking once again myself. The several months that I had spent not smoking prior to this would not be in vain, however, as it would be one of a great many efforts at quitting smoking which would prepare me for my eventual ability to stop smoking altogether. My ultimate triumph over this addiction would not take place for many more years in the future, though.

The primary duty I had as a student intern was facilitating group sessions. The program consisted of a therapist with a master's degree, a

Rehabilitative Coordinator, who had a bachelor's degree in a helping profession, as well as two van drivers. We took turns encouraging group discussions with the clients. These discussions varied in subject matter, but mostly consisted of skills training for coping with symptoms of serious mental illnesses.

Up to this point, I had never led any sort of group discussion, and now I was in a "sink or swim" situation. I had to learn rapidly how to navigate the group dynamics of people with as many differences as they had similarities.

I always envisioned myself as an individual therapist, and felt much more equipped to work with people one-on-one. I soon learned, though, that being able to facilitate a group therapy session was as important a skill as any I needed to acquire if I were to become an effective psychotherapist.

With practice, my proficiency in this area increased, and I felt that I became a much more competent and well-rounded communicator because of my steady practice at this important discipline.

I continued visits to my grandmother throughout this time, describing in glowing terms everything in which I was involved. She was pleased that I finally seemed to be finding my path in the world, and she at one point proudly told one of the nurses who assisted her that I was her egghead.

It was thrilling that she was able to witness me living my dreams, and I beamed when she showed me a picture illustrating a picture of the cleaning products Pride and Joy, saying that I was her own pride and joy.

My studies at school progressed steadily, and I was delighted to finally have access to the textbooks and research related specifically to psychotherapy. An entire new world opened up for me as I studied specific psychotherapeutic techniques and treatment modalities. I poured myself into this work, since I wanted desperately to help other people in the same way I had been helped.

I began comparing the information about psychotherapy I learned to specific things my therapists had said to me over the years, and found myself thinking, "Ah, this is why she said this to me at that time, and that's why she said that to me at another time."

I was still a student though, and had yet to try actually providing therapy to another individual. To some degree, I was insecure about being able to put my knowledge into actual practice, and my own experiences with mental illness did little to alleviate this uncertainty. Part of my field practicum experience meant that I had to spend a certain amount of time with an actual practicing social worker at DMCC. As I sat in on some sessions with one named Nancy, hearing a seasoned therapist at work, I thought to myself, "Wow, I certainly hope I can be as creative and effective as she."

Time passed as I continued my struggle to maintain my working relationship with clients and staff, my grade point average, and a steady diet. One day, as the semester was nearing to a close, I was called into a meeting with my boss, Trish, and Gloria, the clinical director who had conducted my initial interview. They wanted to know if I was interested in a paying job at the MHCNCA.

"Yes," I said. "A job in a mental health facility has been a long-standing dream of mine."

They explained that for the next semester, I could do my internship there for twenty hours a week, as well as working an additional ten paid hours a week. Upon graduation at the end of that semester, I would be hired full time to be a second psychotherapist within the Day Treatment program, with Trish as the other therapist. She would remain the coordinator of the program, and my boss.

I instantly agreed to their terms, feeling overjoyed by the fact that I had finally been offered the career of my dreams. The best part was that I would also be working a short distance away from my grandmother. I even began thinking of ways to move Grandmother to Decatur, since I had been able to see all of the nursing homes in Decatur during my work with The Department of Human Resources. I thought of one that would be perfect for her.

As soon as possible, I told my grandmother that I had actually been offered my dream job, and she shared my moment of happiness. I informed the other social work students of my job offer, and it turned out I was actually the first of the students graduating that year to receive such an offer, knowing where I would be working post-graduation. My life was now definitely on an upward swing, since I had managed to achieve more within the last year and a half than I had dreamed possible in a very long time.

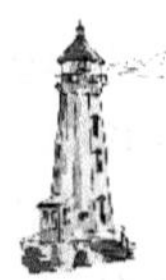

PARTING WAYS

Once I became an official employee, I did a great deal of van driving and had the opportunity to explore throughout Morgan County. I drove through the town and the country, depending upon my route, and it was quite enthralling for me to see cows, horses, and all manner of farm animals on my country drives. Both the clients and staff at DMCC made me feel at home, and my relationships there continued to flourish.

During this time, I made the decision to renew communication with my stepfather, who had been such an important influence throughout my life. With trepidation, I telephoned him one afternoon, hoping he would be willing to talk to me after a two-year silence. He was very receptive to talking, but what he feared when I called was that I was calling to tell him that grandmother's health had declined drastically, or that she had passed away. I quickly told him that she was doing fine, and began to describe to him, in detail, all of the decisions I had made—the events that had occurred, and that I was expected to begin my new profession in a matter of months.

He seemed pleased by this prospect, and happy to know that my life had taken such a positive turn. I let him know how much his influence had affected me and informed him that I had not spoken to him primarily because of the shame I felt for how my life had turned out prior to answering my calling. He seemed to understand this, although it was clear to me, as I am sure it was to him, that our decision to not communicate until now had only resulted in the waste of precious time, time that we could have spent being in touch with one another. I resolved not to let that state of affairs continue, and we maintained contact with one another by telephone and through typed letters sent through the post office, since he was off-line and had no email. He began sending me letters, similar to the ones he sent to Grandmother, that contained a variety of subject matter, including his views of the world.

It was at this time that I met a key individual in my life, and I met her, of all places, on the job at Day Treatment. Eleanor was getting ready to graduate from Athens State University, with a bachelor's degree in Behavioral Science, and she was doing an internship in the Day Treatment Program. We found that we had much in common, and it was not long before we began a genuine friendship. We talked on the telephone quite often, learning more about each other. After a couple months, I asked her to attend the ceremony for the annual induction of candidates into Phi Alpha, the Social Work Honor Society, of which I was already a member.

This ceremony took place in one of the larger rooms on the A&M campus and was quite a dignified ceremony in its symbolism. White candle wax dripped onto my black suit as we held candles to honor the new inductees. Many of my professors and fellow students were interested in meeting the attractive Eleanor, whom I escorted to the event. After the ceremony, we went to one of the Japanese restaurants in Huntsville, called Shogun.

It was not long after this moment that Eleanor and I began dating exclusively, and it was at this point that I confronted the same dilemma I had met before. When should I tell Eleanor about my mental illness, and when she found out, how would she react to it? The fact that we both worked at the same place had the effect of pushing up my decision to inform her far sooner than I likely would have otherwise. I didn't want to take any chances of friction between us at my new job.

So while sitting on the couch in my apartment after one of our first dates, I geared up to tell her about my mental illness, hoping not to see that same sickening expression on her face that I had seen on other occasions when describing my mental health status to girlfriends.

It occurred to me, not for the first time, that it seemed rather unfair that I even had to have these types of conversations that most other people my age didn't have to, while I did not know how she would react and tried to prepare myself for anything. To my grateful surprise, she took the news well and was not overly dismayed by my confession. Her reaction was probably due to the fact that her mother had been struggling with depression for much of her life.

Our relationship endured, and it felt quite refreshing to me that Eleanor knew the truth about me as soon as she did, and that she went against the social tide and accepted me for who I was. She also agreed to keep my secret, and remained the only person from my new working world who was aware that I had a psychotic disorder; and to her credit, she remained true to her word.

I continued to apply myself to my studies, honing my knowledge of ways to provide effective group and individual therapy while trying to apply these techniques to my work at the mental health center, even though I was not technically providing either group or individual therapy, since I had not yet graduated.

With about six weeks to go before graduation and my entry into my new profession, I was studying for the comprehensive final examination, set to take place in a few days' time. That's when I received a fateful telephone call.

My grandmother's friend, Samantha, telephoned me to tell me that my grandmother, Colice, had been taken to the emergency room after experiencing stomach problems. I raced down to the emergency room where I found my grandmother lying on a hospital pallet. I sat with her all that afternoon, awaiting the results of the tests they had run. And after some hours, they said she was free to go and that she had just had a stomach virus of some kind. She was transported back to the nursing home by ambulance, and I met her there much elated that she had nothing to worry about.

A day later, though, Grandmother was back in the hospital. When I got to there, I learned that the situation was much more severe than had originally been suspected.

Grandmother had diverticulitis, and she was placed in the intensive care unit. I telephoned my stepfather with the news he was hoping not to hear when I had phoned him before. For the next six weeks, I was on an emotional rollercoaster, as Grandmother's condition improved and declined with no pattern.

I never knew what to expect. One day she would be unconscious with tubes down her throat, and the next she would be talking to me as if everything was going to be just fine. I spent many hours at the hospital, telling her everything I could think to say to her, never knowing if these would be the last words I was able to say to her or if she were going to make a complete recovery. I continued to balance work and school with my steady visits to the hospital, not knowing if I should postpone my graduation for another year or not.

While weighing my options, I turned to Bernice, my therapist, whose opinion I respected enormously.

When I explained the situation and posed the question of whether I should postpone my graduation, leaning more toward not doing so, as the clients and staff in Day Treatment were counting on me to be there for them upon graduation, she said emphatically, "Don't you do it!"

It was at that point that I realized that it was not just the clients and staff at my new job who were counting on me to hang in there, it was all of the people at the mental health center in my hometown, as well, who realized what I was doing and were encouraged by it.

My future, I realized, was larger than just me, my personal desires, and even my own family. There were so many people counting on me to beat the odds; even my grandmother, who I felt would certainly want me to continue with school, if she were in a clear frame of mind. I could not let them all down.

After about a month of the triple pressure of hospital visits, school, and work, my mind began to do what I have described before: fading out. I was breaking down, as I began to lose concentration and focus. I found myself driving in circles as I was searching for the highway exit to take me to Decatur, a road that I had traveled a hundred times before. My mind felt like it was bleeding inside as I tried to make one concept connect to another one in my efforts to write my final research papers to finish up the work for my master's degree.

As it began to seem less and less likely that my grandmother was going to pull through her illness, I began to see her apparition appear to me at night as I was nearing sleep. My grandmother's image cried out to me in anguish, beckoning me back to her side.

At the hospital, I was only allowed to visit Grandmother during certain hours of the day. The time I couldn't spend visiting, I spent studying. Ironically, I was assigned, at the time, to do research on grief counseling. I found a small hardback book with a jet-black cover on that topic at the mental health center in Decatur. It was with sadness that I carried this book with me on my visits to my grandmother at the hospital. The volume's hardbound cover seemed to mesh to my hand as if it were some sacred text while I paced the hospital's seemingly endless array of lobbies.

Grandmother's relatives began to trickle into Huntsville as they thought this could be the last time they saw this graceful woman, who had touched everyone's life with whom she came in contact. We were all holding on to the slight hope that she could pull through this illness, but we understood that the chances were not good. I realized then that I had better find Bert so that he could say any final words to Grandmother, before she passed away. I went to the restaurant where Bert was washing dishes, and someone showed me to the apartment across the street where he lived.

These were the same apartments where my grandmother and I had lived from 1985 to 1987, before moving to the townhouse. When I located Bert at the apartment complex, it was obvious to me, at any rate, that he was experiencing moderate psychotic symptoms. He appeared to be responding to the internal stimuli of audible hallucinations the whole time I spoke to him.

He told me that he would have to move out of the apartments soon, since he had lost his job at the restaurant and didn't know where he would move next.

Bert had not seen Grandmother since the incident when his psychotic symptoms had caused him to be forcibly removed from the townhouse and hospitalized. I took Bert to the hospital so that he could visit Grandmother. At that time, she had tubes going down her throat. Bert came in crying, much as I had done on a similar visit when I thought she was not going to pull through, but she had made a miraculous recovery.

Grandmother quickly motioned with her hand that she wanted Bert to leave, since his crying was making her feel agitated, and he did.

I questioned Bert, trying to find out if he was willing to accept the truth of his mental illness and ready to be more compliant with treatment, and he indicated that he was not.

I saw nothing I could do for him at that time, especially because my position with the mental health center was tenuous at best. Bert was disappointed by Grandmother's reaction to his presence there.

What Bert didn't know, though, was that while he and Grandmother had grown so distant since his fall from her grace three years earlier, a year or so before his hospitalization occurred, Grandmother had made me promise what I considered at the time a rather curious thing: she wanted me to promise her that I would do everything I could to take care of Bert after she passed away. This seemed like a very odd request at the time, since I was struggling so much with my own identity and trying to figure out what I should do with my own life, even whether to live or die.

Grandmother must have had some kind of premonition of my eventual success, or she was simply a better judge of people than most who knew me. In any event, I had promised that I would do as she requested, if able to do so.

Now, on the verge of graduation, was certainly not a point in time in which fate would yet see my promise fulfilled, and I said my farewells to Bert, gearing up to face another grueling day of triple duty.

Samantha and I celebrated Grandmother Colice's eighty-eighth birthday with her, with tubes down her throat, although she was still conscious.

When the tubes were removed shortly after, and I had one of my few remaining conversations with her, she confessed to me that she was angry with me for trying to take my own life years before. She began to weep, her tears spilling down on her hospital pillow just thinking about it.

It was at that moment that the full ramifications of what I had tried to do hit home, and I realized that in my irrational state of sorrow, I had failed to fully consider how my suicide would have affected the person I loved most in the world.

I could have tried to explain the depthless sorrow and lack of will which drowned my thought processes so many years ago when I attempted suicide. I could have told her that the desire to escape my life on earth was so intense that it felt almost as if I had no control over my own actions. I didn't think she would be able to understand it, though, especially while she was fighting so mightily to hang on to her own life. Instead, I simply acknowledged her feelings, allowing her to tell me what she must have wanted to say to me for the past eight years.

Little did I know though, that other horrors were yet in store for us. In the last week of Grandmother's life, she was often in intense pain and cried out in anguish as I, along with the medical staff and Grandmother's loved ones, could do nothing but watch in heartbreak.

Some older friends of the family who were present gave me a look that told me that they had witnessed such sights before. I had never seen anything like this, and was horror stricken at seeing my grandmother in agony. Thankfully, Grandmother was not in pain the entire time, though, and I continued telling her all of the things I wished to express before she passed.

During this time, I had no idea how long Grandmother would continue living, and my colleagues at work and school were just as baffled as I was, as Grandmother's chances of survival waxed and waned over a six-week period of time.

Ironically, I was heavy-hearted as I attended my graduation at the A&M stadium, where the world seemed a surreal mix of tragedy and triumph. Friends came to witness the realization of my dream, though the reality of my world, with my grandmother, seemed more like a nightmare.

After graduation, I raced to show my grandmother my diploma and watched with awe as she brushed her fingers over its coarse leather hide. She had lived to see the realization of my dream and hers. She had always told me she wanted to live long enough to see me graduate, and she had managed to live long enough to see me earn not one, but three diplomas. That night I kneeled down on the floor of my apartment and gave thanks to God for allowing me to overcome the obstacles I had, to reach my dream. While I was doing this, I was surprised when all of the lights went out in the neighborhood. I continued to pray in the dark to my heavenly Father to alleviate my grandmother's suffering, and to give me the strength I needed to continue my life's journey.

Three days later, Grandmother Colice was gone from this world, although her spirit remains with me for life. Bernice consoled me on my loss, as I cried bitter tears for losing the physical presence of the person I cherished above all others. She was closer to me than any other human being had ever been. I realized that I was lucky for having known her for the time that I had, but this did little to assuage the grief.

Grandmother had a wealthy cousin, named Pete, who paid for all of her funeral arrangements, since I was still virtually penniless.

At the funeral, I wore the same black suit that I had worn to my induction into the Social Work Honor Society, Phi Alpha, three months earlier. I had been unable to entirely remove the candle wax, and felt a tinge of self-consciousness at this.

Eleanor was unable to attend the funeral with me, since she was with her family in Florida, on vacation. They had asked me to go with them, but I was unable to join them, not knowing how long my grandmother might live.

My friend Sabrina attended the funeral though, along with scores of friends who had known me throughout my life with Grandmother. Other attendees were family members of ours from other states. What I discovered to my shock, was that the funeral actually seemed to break into two factions.

One faction consisted of people who had known me throughout my life with Grandmother, and who were there to comfort me, as well as to pay homage to my grandmother. Other attendees seemed somewhat resentful of me, and were there to comfort Samantha, who had provided care for Grandmother for the last few years of her life. These family members included my uncle's sons from Texas, one a district judge and one a federal assistant district attorney. They greeted me very curtly and made no further efforts to speak to me at all during the ceremony. Instead they spent their time and energy doting on Samantha, who was clearly upset. At one point my adopted sister Kim, who was present at the funeral, even exchanged angry words with Samantha, though I don't know exactly what was said.

I still do not fully understand why matters turned out the way they did at the funeral. I don't know if it was the stigma of my mental illness, or if my very existence represented for them some notion of family dishonor, since my father was not present in my life. Perhaps my relatives from Texas were still angry over the scathing letter my stepfather had written them, asking them for help. Or maybe it was a combination of all those things. In any event, the way things turned out was something my own experience had not prepared me for in any way, and I was certainly surprised by it all.

Perhaps the fact that Grandmother had been such a major influence in the lives of all these people meant that such infighting during her memorial was inevitable. That I was the ultimate heir, as her adopted son, of such dignity and grace, was not a fact that was lost on me, but one that left me with a profound sense of awe.

I had gotten in touch with the new minister of the First Baptist Church, of which my grandmother was the oldest living member, who agreed to deliver Grandmother's eulogy. He recited the Psalm, which I knew to be her favorite, the 23rd. He also read a poem she had always told me she wanted to be read at her funeral: Tennyson's "Crossing the Bar." At my insistence, the minister also read Matthew 6:26, which says, "See the birds of the sky, that they don't sow, neither do they reap, nor gather into barns. Your heavenly Father feeds them. Aren't you of much more value than they?"

When the funeral ended, I made my farewells to all of the people who were interested in speaking with me. The others drove off to participate in their own mourning meals. After the funeral, I drove to DMCC, still wearing my black suit with the slight stain of candle wax, and described to Trish and Mike all that had happened.

It is an interesting feeling to be loved and respected by many people while being despised and rejected by others. Perhaps this is part of the human condition, though as I ponder on it further, I realize that I never met anyone who did not share a love for my grandmother after meeting her.

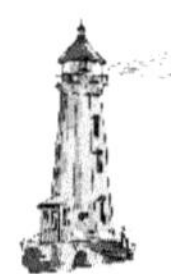

SHAKE UP

I continued my yearlong daily commute from Huntsville to Decatur; although now, I was traveling to work full-time, as a psychotherapist. I was still in a state of shock from the loss of my grandmother. This was especially poignant because her death had occurred at a moment that otherwise would have been one of pure elation.

I continued to see my therapist, Bernice, despite the fact that I now had Blue Cross insurance, and opportunities to gain access to mental health care at other facilities. The HMCMHC had done so much for me already that I found it hard to imagine receiving higher quality services anywhere else. A new young doctor had begun working at the HMCMHC, and my therapist introduced me to him, telling him that I now had my MSW.

The young doctor then looked at me with a solemn gaze and said to me, "You give us all hope!"

I was not expecting that sort of response from the young doctor and was somewhat taken aback by it. I found that it did give me a certain thrill to hear him say that. I was certainly pleased that my success had this effect upon people interested in the welfare of my population, as a whole. I felt thankful that I could be a focal point of the shared hope and celebration of consumers, their families, and mental health professionals alike. I also realized instantly that it was very important that I remain humble in the face of such high praise.

I had seen too many tragic circumstances in my life and the lives of those I cared about to let myself be thrown off balance by concentrating on my own accomplishments. I had enjoyed the help of a great many people throughout my life to make it as far as I had. I did not want to allow pride to make me lose sight of such an important truth. My calling was to serve others through my experiences, knowledge, and compassion. Reveling in my own accomplishments would be contrary to my primary objective.

Now that I was a therapist at DMCC, I had to focus my mind on learning the practical aspects of how to work at a very stressful job. The paperwork demands alone were enormous. I had to thoroughly train my mind in the discipline of staying on top of these responsibilities.

Up to this point, I had yet to actually have a therapy session with a client. My fear was that I would not know how to respond to what my clients would tell me about their problems. When I was thrust full swing into this responsibility, I was thankful to discover that the words I needed in order to assist my new clients came readily to my lips.

Having been the recipient of therapy for the past eight years, I found myself repeating some of the phrases my own therapists had said to me. The training I had received in school also gave me proper insight into how to conduct an individual therapy session. My own experiences as a consumer only enhanced my ability to relate to my clients and help them find the right solutions for the problems they were facing.

Dealing with people, as complicated as they can be, was an enormous challenge. There were a thousand demands from a thousand different voices, and all of them urgent. I was very fortunate; I had Trish to train me for my new job. She had the patience, firmness, and supportive nature necessary to train me effectively.

I read in one of my social work textbooks that it was important for a social worker to live in whatever community he or she was serving, if at all possible. This made practical sense to me, both personally and professionally. Though I was still grateful for the apartment which had provided me shelter at a time when I was in desperate need, the yearning desire I had to escape its impoverished confines was stronger than ever. I now had more resources than I'd ever had in my life, making such a move possible.

My new romantic interest, Eleanor, who lived in Decatur, introduced me to an apartment manager who was the proprietor of the place where she and one of her girlfriends had lived for a time, and I soon arranged to move there. The apartment I moved into was just as modest as the one I was leaving, except that it had two bedrooms, instead of one.

Eleanor's father allowed me to borrow his pickup truck for the move, which took several trips. He was the principal of the Developmental School in Decatur, which he'd founded upon his return from Vietnam. This school provided education for children with intellectual disabilities.

During my move from Huntsville to Decatur, a rather interesting encounter, and one I did not feel quite prepared for, occurred. Eleanor and I were outside of my old apartment in Huntsville, loading some things into the truck, when Bert suddenly appeared.

He was clearly in a more psychotic state than he was the last time I saw him, and he was eager to show me a non-permanent Spiderman tattoo he had on his forearm. Eleanor had never met Bert, and I didn't quite know how to handle the situation. I was concerned about her reaction to him.

"It looks like you're moving," he beamed, while his eyes seemed to be staring at something a million miles away.

"Yes," I said. "I'm moving to Decatur." After a long pause I said, "That way I can be closer to my job."

"Oh you got a new job?" he asked.

"Yes." I answered. "Don't you remember I told you I was about to start a new job as a therapist, when I spoke to you at your apartment, about Grandma?"

"Oh, I remember now." He said continuing to have that strange smile lighting up his face. Then the smile suddenly vanished, "That sure was sad about grandma."

"Yes…yes it was really horrible!" I said.

I made sure that Bert had my cell phone number, and then I ushered Eleanor away from the surprising meeting, relieved that Bert could not just appear in a psychotic state at the door of my new apartment in Decatur. Eleanor was very gracious about the situation, and I was happy to see that she didn't seem to have a negative reaction to meeting my brother.

I hadn't told Bert about Grandmother's funeral, and felt somewhat justified for that difficult decision as I saw Bert in his current psychotic state. Grandmother's funeral was stressful enough as it was without me having to worry about Bert having a psychotic reaction.

I was certain that Bert was still unwilling to accept mental health treatment. I resolved to try to help him whenever I was in a position to do so, and whenever Bert was ready to receive the assistance I could offer.

Being a therapist is a very demanding profession, even for a person who does not have a serious mental illness. Based on what I can gather from the experiences of other therapists and my knowledge of other professions, it ranks with about the most demanding and difficult work a person can do, and it certainly didn't take me very long to figure this out. Despite the difficulty of the course I had chosen, I remained determined to be a therapist.

One of my responsibilities as a therapist that I particularly enjoyed, was the opportunity I had to shape young minds newly diagnosed with serious mental illness. I wanted to be as effective in treating these young souls as my therapist, Marilyn, had been with me.

Invariably, they were in denial about what had happened to them—as I had been—so that most of what I said to them would not really make an enormous impact until a few months, or a year down the road. Unlike other new therapists, though, I knew that this would be the case, and was spared the sense of disappointment that my first therapist, Marilyn, must have felt when I had a second relapse of symptoms.

I was thrilled at the notion that I was in a position to genuinely help these people overcome the enormous obstacles they were facing. My experience as a Consumer of Mental Health Services was invaluable in this context, since I was able to provide information to clients that was invaluable to their recovery. At the same time, I buffered my sense of grief at their loss with the knowledge that I could help them along their own road to recovery.

I was an expert in a subject about which they knew nothing, but would need to know in order to carry on with their lives. In my mind, no one else was in a better position than I to provide these young people the knowledge they so desperately needed. I knew from my experience that the gratification of seeing one in recovery from his or her serious mental illness was not instantaneous. I was happy, nonetheless, knowing that my words were making a profound impact on their lives.

My eventual goal was to become a psychotherapist in outpatient services, where the two therapists I had worked with at the HMCMHC had worked, and I had confidence that I would reach that goal.

As the months of work passed, my confidence that no one there knew about my past history of mental illness began to unravel. One incident in particular began a chain reaction in my mind, in which I became unsure of what my coworkers really did or didn't know about my mental health status. It was around Christmas—the first hard Christmas, because Grandmother was not there to celebrate with me. There was a small party held for the Board Members of the MHCNCA. The Board was the body who set policy for the organization, and to whom the Director of the MHCNCA, Marie Hood, answered directly.

Marie Hood was a formidable woman in her own right, who managed to fulfill her numerous duties as Director for a vast organization while living with the crippling physical disability, muscular sclerosis. People in mental health circles revered her.

I walked into the party, which was held in one of the large group rooms at DMCC and had settled down with a nice plate of finger foods when something unexpected happened. Doris Todd, one of the board members was introduced to me and, as it turned out, she had been an active member of NAMI, Huntsville, and had known me for a long time in my role as a volunteer and as a member.

My conviction that my past was completely unknown was shattered into a thousand pieces in that moment, and I quickly fled the room, feeling agitated that my new world might be in jeopardy. Trish could see that I was upset, as I must have looked like I had seen a ghost. I did all that I could to maintain a semblance of composure, hoping that no mention would be made of my past.

My natural fears, amplified in people with my particular disorder, remained set in place as I became increasingly convinced that everyone I worked with now knew the truth about my disability. When I heard subtle innuendos or slight nuances in speech from coworkers, I convinced myself that these were somehow related to me and my mental illness. This was not the case though, as I discovered after receiving a shocking phone call.

Peggy, the long-standing head of human resources telephoned me and said that Social Security had called her asking all kinds of questions about my income, and she wanted to know what I wanted her to be able to tell them. I was shocked that the SSA had telephoned her at all, especially since I supplied the SSA with all the information that they wanted and had made specific requests to them not to contact my employer in any way.

With no other explanation available, I told Peggy to provide the SSA any information they requested, and ended the telephone conversation in as graceful a manner as I could.

After many minutes of careful—if fretful—consideration, I concluded that the best thing for me to do was to tell Trish everything about my disability and my past. I felt it would be best to have my employer know the entirety of my situation, as opposed to having lingering questions about why the SSA was making inquiries about me.

I told Trish that I needed to speak to her about something and then screwed up my courage to tell her the full truth about my life as a PLMI. Despite my nagging concern that everyone knew about my mental illness already, Trish was shocked to hear my revelation. She convinced me to tell our supervisor, Mike, about the situation, and I sat down with him to do just that.

He had been equally oblivious to the fact that I had schizophrenia, and seemed just as surprised as Trish. Not only was I wrong about thinking that they might somehow already know that I had a mental illness, but I was also incorrect in my fears that something dire might happen in terms of my employment situation, were they to find out. They took this knowledge in stride, and nothing really changed.

After a month or so, I learned that Trish had taken another position within the organization and was now to be a psychotherapist in the geriatrics program in the neighboring town of Athens. I was sad to see Trish go, and appreciative for all of the help and guidance she had provided me over the year and a half that I had known her.

Her departure meant that I would be working with a new clinician who would take her place as the Day Treatment Coordinator. The man who took her place was Kenny, a man in his early fifties, who was a seasoned clinician. I learned a great deal from Kenny, who seemed to have an almost magical rapport with the clients.

He played a guitar and would serenade the clients with wonderful melodies on our fun days. Kenny taught me many things, both in terms of paperwork and in how to engage the clients. Many of the things he taught me, however, I did not realize until after he departed the program. That was within about five months when he took a job at, of all places, the HMCMHC, the place where I continued to receive mental health services.

Kenny's departure meant that I would be working with a new clinician at the helm of the Day Treatment program. Her name was Carmen, and she had considerable experience as a therapist, as well as her own ideas about how to improve the Day Treatment program. Carmen was an attractive lady, close to my age, who had an incredible amount of energy. As it turned out, she was related to Samantha, the lady who had provided such good care for Grandmother at Windsor House and seemed to share the same quality of an inexhaustible supply of energy and enthusiasm.

By this time, Eleanor and I had become engaged. There was surprisingly little romantic pomp and circumstance involved in my "popping the question." We had been in discussion about this for some time.

It basically involved me giving Eleanor one of the few remaining possessions I had of my grandmother's: the engagement ring she always wore on her hand. The ring was from the nineteen thirties, and had a unique design, which Eleanor appreciated.

Eleanor accepted the ring, and we made plans to move into a house of our own. After working with a real estate agent, we found the perfect home; and on Valentine's Day 2005, we bought our first house.

I made another trip to Talladega to attend another Consumer Conference. Ironically though, this time I was going there as a staff member to assist consumers from Decatur, making the trip on busses chartered by the MHCNCA. Linda Pierce, a charismatic and long-standing case manager, asked me to assist her as the male staff member. I had managed to walk a fine line by not allowing my identity as a consumer to be known to my clients, although this situation tested my capacity for maintaining my privacy to its limit.

If the clients I traveled there with, or Linda, were wondering how I seemed to know so many of the people there, particularly the ones from Huntsville, they didn't acknowledge their curiosity.

It was a spectacular experience to get to see so many of my old friends in the conference atmosphere, because they could see that I was doing well.

I had a deep respect for these people who had survived so much, and I cared deeply about their opinion of me. I realized that advances in medication, and in the mental health system as a whole, had much to do with the fact that I was now able to accomplish dreams that must have seemed out of reach to them. In a way, I saw their presence in my life as much like seeing my ancestors.

My friends from Huntsville spoke about Our Place, the Consumer Run Drop-in Center, which remained active, providing an assortment of activities for its members.

In my relationships with my old friends, I was as a child adopted into their family. In my relationship with clients, I had to be the authority figure, no matter their age or level of experience. Their lives, and quality of life, in so many instances, rested on my shoulders.

In my role as a therapist, I had to decide whose thoughts were suicidal enough to require hospitalization. My personal experiences gave me a natural edge that is difficult to describe. I was near enough to death in my own contemplation of suicide that I had developed a knack for determining how close others are to their own self-destruction.

Mary Reeder, who continued to pour her considerable powers into the maintenance and expansion of Our Place, received the RESPECT award that year, and I congratulated her profusely for this honor. The RESPECT award is given by consumers in Alabama to people who have worked diligently for the betterment of the lives of PLMI. It is the highest honor one can earn in the world of mental health in Alabama.

QUESTION MARK

Opportunity knocked on my door in a way that I did not expect when I spoke to my friend Cherie. She worked on the other side of the building in the Quest program, which provided substance abuse counseling to People Living with Addictions (PLA). What Cherie asked was whether or not I would be interested in applying for a job opening, which had become available in that program.

I thanked Cherie for telling me about this opportunity, and said that I would certainly consider the idea. It was August, 2005; I was almost thirty-one years old, and I had been a therapist in the Day Treatment program for one year and three months. I was excited by the prospect of gaining additional experience in becoming as effective a therapist as I could possibly be, and I knew that learning everything I could about treating addiction would be an important addition to my palette of mental health knowledge.

While the prospect of accepting a position in another branch of mental health service provision might seem at odds with my ultimate goal of becoming a therapist in the outpatient program, I thought there was no conflict.

Those with mental illnesses like schizophrenia, bipolar disorder, or major depression, often struggled with co-occurring addictions. The story of Bert is inextricably threaded throughout this personal journey, and brings this reality to light better than any other example.

I had received an unexpected telephone call from Bert a few weeks before this. He told me that he was working in a factory in the neighboring town of Madison, had an apartment and a car, and wanted me to know that he was doing well. I asked him if he was taking his medication for mental health, feeling all the while that I already knew the answer.

I was not surprised to find out that he was not on his medication. I had seen this pattern before: Bert rising from the ashes, only to collapse once again into the heap of psychotic symptoms and addiction. I'd observed the tragedy more times than I felt I was able to bear. I told Bert that there was really nothing else for us to talk about.

In retrospect, I was not pleased with how I handled this situation. My instinct for survival trumped my feelings of familial obligation in this instance, and my own fallibility as a human being was never more obvious.

I sat down with my supervisor, Mike, to ask for his guidance in my decision to apply for the position as a substance abuse counselor. He encouraged me to make the move to Quest. He had worked there before, and had much insight into what it would be like to provide services in that arena. With high hopes, I met with Cathy Goodwin, the Program Director of Quest, to discuss a possible transfer to the Quest Intensive Outpatient Program. She seemed pleased during our interview to hear that my desire to help PLA was genuine.

Addiction is a type of mental illness, categorized as any other type of mental health diagnosis. It differs in that it is not considered a Serious Mental Illness (SMI), such as schizophrenia or major depression, though its symptoms can create as many problems for people who live with these disorders, as well as their families.

The stigma attached to this population is great, and compounded, because many people attribute addiction to some kind of moral weakness, as opposed to biological and psychological factors. These factors make recovery from addiction a difficult transformation to undergo and maintain.

I realized that people living with co-occurring SMI and addiction comprised a large percentage of the people receiving mental health treatment. I thought that with my experience I could become an effective tool for treating both conditions simultaneously.

I felt empowered by Cathy's obvious acceptance of my mental illness. Her faith in my ability to master other disciplines, other than treatment of people living with SMI boosted my self-confidence to a new level. She demonstrated her confidence by reminding me that I had worked with DHR before I had ever worked in the Day Treatment

Program, and should not feel limited in the type of service I could provide as a helping professional.

After an enormous amount of soul searching, I accepted the transfer from the Day Treatment program to Quest. I then had to make this decision clear to the clients in the Day Treatment program. I explained to them that this was an opportunity for me to increase my understanding of how to better serve my clients. While sad to see my departure, they understood that I was making what I thought was the right move.

When I started my new job, I soon learned that many of the images I had of PLA were completely distorted. I discovered that these people were both kind and generous to one another, when not confronted with their own addictions. They were, for the most part, working hard at full-time jobs, and were not the homeless people at the end of their rope that I had imagined them to be. In essence, they were pretty much like most people in society, except that they had addictions which created enough complications in their lives that they sought treatment.

Some of my new clients criticized me for the fact that I was not in recovery from an addiction of my own. They did not know that I was living in recovery from a mental illness at least as devastating as theirs, an essential component of my ability to treat them. It allowed me, to a large degree, to empathize with what they were experiencing.

When I discussed with my own therapist, Bernice, that I would become a substance abuse counselor, she supported my decision. In fact, she confided that she had been a substance abuse counselor for about five years. She said that some of her clients had given her a hard time about not being in recovery from an addiction. She reinforced my understanding that one did not have to experience the exact same challenges in order to effectively help another to overcome their obstacles.

This is not to say that I do not value the experiences of people in recovery from addictions in helping other people recover. Treating other people with psychotic disorders in Day Treatment taught me that my own experience with recovery was one of the most powerful tools I had. My experiences as a Consumer of Mental Health Services made it easier for me to treat others experiencing similar symptoms. I intended to prove, though, that I could be an effective substance abuse counselor, despite any lack of personal experience with serious addiction.

In the run-up to my wedding, I began to reflect on my past. I had spent year after lonely year apart from much of the larger community. My solitude began in childhood and persisted, despite my best efforts, throughout my adolescence and into adulthood. It always felt as if human companionship was just within reach until some upsetting tragedy or life upheaval would propel me further away from the camaraderie I sought.

It always seemed that there was the proverbial "light at the end of the tunnel," but as the years stretched on, it often felt as if the tunnel grew longer and narrower, until eventually it felt as if the tunnel was so narrow that it was choking the life out of me. I often heard songs on the radio that were odes to loneliness, and I wondered what these songwriters must have experienced to allow them to create such meaningful melodies and lyrics about the topic. I wondered how they could get things so right when it seemed so unlikely that they had experienced loneliness on such a scale as I had, lasting year after year.

One result of this aspect of my life was that I had grown conditioned to finding enjoyment in my own company. It also meant that I had a world of knowledge to gain about interacting successfully with other people, and certainly a lot to learn about maintaining a marriage.

Loneliness is like poverty, in many ways. While you may be extremely lonely, like someone may be extremely poor, it seems that there are always more people out there who are more lonely or poorer than you are. As a therapist, I have certainly encountered people who were lonelier than I ever thought about being. One grows accustomed to living a life of isolation, similar to the way one can learn to live on a very tight budget.

As a psychotherapist, I spent a great amount of time prodding people out of their isolation.

"The only way you can break out of this cycle, is to make yourself seek other people to socialize with, even though you may not feel like it at first," I told them. "In time, you will discover that there is a whole part of your life involving others that you have been missing."

The groom's party for our wedding consisted of three men. My best man was David, who had been like a brother throughout my life. Tommy was also in the groom's party. The other man in the groom's party was Eleanor's brother, Mack.

The site of the rehearsal dinner was in what had to be one of the oldest houses in Decatur. The creaky floorboards and fanciful decorations gave the distinct air of an old funhouse one would find at a county fair. This whimsical feel made me think of my grandmother and of all the good times that I experienced under her roof. In all my happiness, I was sad that Grandmother wouldn't see my wedding.

Eleanor's maternal grandparents had passed away a year or so before we met, and I know that they were very much on the minds of Eleanor and her family.

One addition to our wedding—the idea of my Mother-in-law, to be—was to have two vases standing near the altar. These represented the presence of both my mother and my grandmother. After much stress and many dinners, we finally said our vows in front of God and man on December 2nd, 2005. We then watched all of the guests proceed back to the ancient house where we'd had our rehearsal dinner.

Eleanor and I soon discovered that the bride and groom rarely take part in all of the sumptuous refreshments which the guests enjoy, as we made our best efforts to speak to everyone who had taken part in our wedding ceremony. Speeches were given, and then I raised a wine glass to my lips and took a sip.

An observer might find it somewhat hypocritical that I was still a social drinker, though my occupation consisted of helping other people come to grips with their addictions and I was in recovery from SMI; and to some degree, he or she would be correct. It was certainly unwise for me to continue to drink, even on a social basis.

My life was going well enough for me that I thought that drinking small amounts of alcohol was something I could handle. Over time, I would come to learn that it was necessary for me to abstain from alcohol altogether. I eventually realized that consuming even small amounts of alcohol made it more difficult for me to manage all of my symptoms. I found that my ability to concentrate was broken less often when I finally learned to quit drinking. This realization grew in fits and starts, though. I might not drink anything for one year and then drink on two or three occasions the next. The net result, though, was that I drank less and less over time, until I ceased drinking altogether.

One part of my wedding celebration that did not involve drinking was put together by Mary Reeder, my old friend. She called me a couple of weeks after my wedding.

She was still working with the CMHS in Madison County, operating Our Place. She invited Eleanor and me to a party celebrating our nuptials; we were happy to go. The drop-in center had really expanded by this time, operating out of their own house where they provided a number of activities for its members to enjoy.

Eleanor and I were pampered by love and affection by Mrs. Reeder and the consumers with whom I had lived and worked for so many years. Mrs. Reeder had prepared beautiful flower arrangements throughout the house, and the weather outside was gorgeous as we celebrated with Our Place.

I was happy about the opportunity to celebrate my wedding with this group of people, and felt in many ways that our marriage had been consecrated, in a unique way, by this event. Mrs. Reeder and other friends from Our Place seemed pleased to meet my new bride.

After our trip to Our Place, the last of the wedding ceremonies were concluded and we began our life as a married couple. Being a married man was certainly a drastic change from the lifestyle I had maintained as a single person. I had to become adjusted to having somebody who was in the same household with me all of the time. Eleanor was good about giving me my personal space, though. Our jobs were both so stressful that we both often needed time alone to decompress from the events of the work day.

Some of my clients had dual diagnoses, which meant that they had both SMI and a substance abuse disorder. Sometimes, clients with whom I had worked in Day Treatment were transferred to Quest if they were experiencing problems related to addictions.

I developed a rather different approach to working with these clients. I quickly discovered that they often felt alienated from the other clients in the Quest Program who were not dually diagnosed. Every now and then, one of the clients without a co-occurring disorder would say something offensive with regard to those with SMI in the group.

Whenever this occurred, I patiently corrected the speaker and did my best to explain the facts about mental illness, including the reality that they had been diagnosed with a mental illness in the form of a substance abuse disorder. They understood once all the facts about mental illness were explained to them. They then made efforts to avoid potentially offensive speech.

I attended Alcoholics Anonymous meetings with my group, on occasion, and learned all that I could about the Twelve Step model and the precepts set in place by Bill Wilson when he wrote the Alcoholics Anonymous Big Book.

I found an abundance of material in his book to draw upon in my efforts to convince people that recovery was a necessary component in their pursuit of a quality life. The Big Book often speaks about the "insanity" of continued substance abuse by PLMI, and it was written long before the American Psychological Association classified substance dependence as a form of mental illness.

Whenever someone completed the Quest program, he or she received a small plastic medallion that looked like a poker chip with the Quest logo on it. These looked similar to the chips people receive at Alcoholics Anonymous. We would end meetings by saying the Serenity Prayer. This prayer is well known in substance abuse recovery circles, and was one I had recited myself at the Consumer Conference in Talladega, as it had been incorporated into the recovery mantra there.

"God grant me the serenity to accept the things I cannot change, the courage to change the things that I can, and the wisdom to know the difference."

These powerful words can help people in recovery from SMI, substance abuse, or both. They can help anyone facing life's inevitable challenges and difficulties.

Life always places obstacles in our path, whether it is the death of a loved one, sickness, or financial stress; these we cannot control. In the face of all this uncertainty, all we can do is manage the situations over which we do have control, in order to reduce the risk of the unknown and to limit its impact upon us when it does occur.

The philosophy and mindset of people in recovery from substance abuse disorders is very much in harmony with people who are in recovery from SMI. Working with my clients in this atmosphere of recovery, I was reminded of my cousin Bill Smith, who'd had such a large hand in my upbringing.

Although Bill passed away when I was twelve years old, he was quite influential as a part of my upbringing. It was Bill's voice that I could hear so clearly in my mind during the events leading to my commitment to the state hospital.

Bill's voice was echoing through my mind and spirit once again, although in a much less audible way, and in a manner that I was better equipped to handle. Bill was a retired Air Force Veteran, a World War II fighter pilot, a successful retired real estate developer, an avid golfer and fisherman, and a devoted church member. But that was not all Bill was.

Bill had been in recovery from alcoholism for the past twenty years when he met me at age seven, and he was a devoted member of Alcoholics Anonymous.

I remember how he proudly showed me the plastic chips of varying solid colors he was awarded for successive years of recovery, and I could imagine, even then, how many people Bill must have helped in their own journey through recovery.

He stressed to me at a very early age how important it was to stay free of addictive substances, and his admonitions lingered in my mind. Bill was, in essence, the archetype for what the people in my care could hope to achieve, and I felt very fortunate to be able to honor his legacy by continuing his quest.

In my work at Quest, I found myself working with people of all education levels, economic levels, and levels of cognitive functioning. What I came to realize was that the disease of addiction does not discriminate. No matter the factors above, nor in race or gender—whether or not one has a disability. Addiction is an equal opportunity destroyer of people's lives, and of the people who care for them.

I might find myself having an individual session with a professor one hour, counseling a grandmother the next hour, and the next speaking to a youth who works at the local grocery. I cared very deeply about whether or not the people in my care continued to be free of drugs and alcohol. That was the most stressful aspect of my job.

Part of successfully finishing Quest meant that those completing it had to be able to pass random drug screens. Additionally, they could have no more than two relapses without adverse consequences. The sanction might be dismissal from the program, or referral to an inpatient facility. Most of the people in my care stood to lose a great deal if they could not successfully graduate from the program. For them, failure might mean losing their jobs, going to jail, or losing custody of their children. It was my responsibility to administer these drug screens, and to try to mete out the consequences of the results in a fair and impartial manner.

Although I was not the final authority regarding the consequences of a failed drug screen, I was the official on the front line to whom those authorities would be listening. I felt the burden as a heavy one, and often found it difficult to provide comfort and assurance to a person one day, only to have to feel like an executioner the next.

I sometimes watched the daytime television show *Judge Mathis,* and found myself thinking about the way he managed to orchestrate the court in a way that was both entertaining to spectators and also demonstrating his authority to make the final decisions. I felt the same way he must have felt on his show, trying to balance appealing to my audience in order to stimulate an interest in recovery, with fairness in exercising authority.

I stayed in regular contact with my stepfather. He was now seventy-eight years old. Much of our communication was in the form of typed letters we sent to one another through standard mail, since he still had an aversion to email. He told me that he was pleased that I had become a proficient writer. We talked on the telephone from time to time as well, although it seemed as if the letters gave us more range in communicating our ideas.

About nine months after our wedding, I went to the mailbox one day and found a letter from St. Louis. This time the letter was not from Dave, but his son, my stepbrother, Wendell. When I opened the letter, I was shocked to read that my stepfather, Dave, had passed. It turned out that he had needed another heart surgery, which he didn't survive. Wendell did not know my telephone number, but had the return address from my letters to tell me the tragic news. He left me his telephone number in the letter.

I called Wendell; I hadn't spoken to him in many years. He was completely devastated by what had happened, as was I. Dave had always maintained an exceptionally healthy lifestyle and had no health problems, other than his heart condition. Wendell told me that Dave had received the last letter I had sent him just before he went in for surgery.

Eleanor and I made plans to fly to St. Louis the next day to attend

Dave's funeral. We realized that Dave had not attended our wedding because he undoubtedly felt stressed about his upcoming surgery, and he may have even sensed that he would be passing on soon.

We made the sad trip to the airport to catch our flight to St. Louis. I had not been on an airplane in more than ten years; my bicycle trip across the country in the summer of 1995 had necessitated a flight to San Francisco. Dave had driven me to the airport in Nashville ten years ago so I could catch my flight. I could still remember Dave sitting in a wheelchair he found at the front of the airport while we awaited my flight. There was something vaguely amusing about seeing him sit in that wheelchair, both of us knowing he was in perfect health. Flying was a different story, post 9/11. I now had to remove my belt in order to make it through security.

I imagine that my stepfather must have felt this feeling of surrealism when he left his home in Huntsville, where he had lived more years than I had been alive, to go back to his previous home in St. Louis.

Wendell had been working for some time now as a consumer bankruptcy attorney and was considered an expert in that specialty. He had been married for many years to his wife, Becky, who had been a paralegal. They worked together as a team in the law firm where Wendell was a partner. I felt very much like a stranger in a strange land as soon as I stepped off the airplane. Wendell and Becky did much to make Eleanor and I feel welcome, making sure that we had lodgings at a nice hotel and buying us dinner at a nice restaurant.

I had recently moved from a mid-sized city to a much smaller city, and I was not used to being in a city as large as St. Louis. With the exception of Andre, one of Dave's older friends from Huntsville, most of the people who attended the funeral were Wendell's friends and associates. Wendell and Becky had managed to create the perfect climate for memorializing a man who had played such an enormous role in both our lives. There were a number of pictures of Dave when he was young. In one of these, he was running alongside a locomotive, and his spirit seemed to soar alongside the great machine.

Like that locomotive, Dave seemed to be the harbinger of a new age. His reason and compassion suggested visions of a world which could be better than the one we now inhabit. Perhaps this was why Dave spent so much time doing volunteer work for the Railroad Museum in

Huntsville. I couldn't help but think about my childhood experience of working as a gofer on the Railroad Museum's steam locomotive as it made its annual excursion to Chattanooga. My grandmother had ridden along, and we explored the grounds of the train depot in Chattanooga together.

Dave was always doing volunteer work in one way or another, and even when he was not he was thinking of new ways to distribute resources to people in need. He had a pen pal in Poland, for instance, who his generosity had enriched at very little expense through small gifts of cash and goods. Dave lived a frugal lifestyle, which allowed him to give donations of money and time to people and institutions that he felt would create greater good in our society.

Classical music, Dave's favorite, played for all of the mourners. The harmonious climate of this funeral stood in stark contrast my grandmother's, which had turned into such a fractious event. The judges that attended Dave's funeral thought very highly of Wendell and treated Eleanor and me with respect.

Bitter tears streamed uncontrollably as I thought of the vast stores of knowledge and kindness which were now gone from this world. But the evidence of his influence was shining in the lives Dave had touched, and in the many works of his hands. Dave was a builder of everything from a model A ford, which he put together from scratch, to the plethora of model planes and trains which he had put together and painted by hand before I was born. Examples of these were on display in his new house, which was like the same cluttered workshop of an ingenious mind that his house in Huntsville had been, but on a slightly smaller scale. A large model train engine was mounted upon his wall the way someone else might mount a giant trout.

After the funeral, we went to the gravesite, a beautiful and ancient place; and as we walked to this site it was bitter cold. It was the first cold day in St. Louis that year and the Missouri wind cut through my black suit like paper and bit deeply into my bones. Dave's older friend, Andre, placed African Violets lovingly on the grave as I wondered how they could possibly survive the biting, chill wind.

Eleanor and I returned to Decatur with heavy hearts, grateful that we had the chance to see my stepfather's final resting place and mourn his passing. Back on the job at Quest, I had to carry on, despite such a heavy personal loss, much the same way as I had when I worked at Day Treatment after the loss of my grandmother. My technique in assisting PLA continually improved as I synthesized my own approach to treating these illnesses.

Marijuana was a drug that I found particularly difficult to convince people was causing them problems. Popular culture in 2006 was busy spreading misinformation about its effects, despite scientific research that clearly demonstrated its harmful properties.

One harmful feature of particular interest to those in the mental health community is its tendency to increase the chances of having a psychotic break with reality in those with a genetic predisposition to experiencing these symptoms in the first place. When people say that marijuana makes them feel "paranoid," this is the effect that they are referring to.

One who has already experienced psychosis should definitely avoid unlocking a plethora of hallucinations and delusions that can accompany marijuana use. The level of THC, the part of the substance that creates the high, has been increased by the plant's producers throughout the years to such an extent that this effect is vastly worse than it was many years ago. While all substances tend to exacerbate mental health symptoms, convincing people that marijuana was dangerous was definitely a challenge.

I would say to my clients, "Let's assume that what you say is true, and that marijuana use really isn't particularly harmful. You still have one enormous problem on your hands, and do you know what that is?"

At this point, I would be met with interested stares, but no answers.

"You still can't pass a drug test! Society, being what it is, has dictated that you will not be eligible for just about any job you apply for if you cannot pass, and continue to pass, drug tests. Marijuana remains in your system longer than any other drug. This means that even if you hit the jackpot, and someone tells you that you can have your dream job and can start work at it right away, and 'all you have to do is pass a drug test,' you will not even have the opportunity to do so."

I would then tell them the story of my time out of work, and my inability to find a job I really wanted.

I would tell them the story of how one day, I was telephoned out of the blue to begin the security job which propelled me out of poverty, leaving out the details about having mental illness.

I told them how the next thing I heard out of my potential employer's mouth was, "You will have to pass a drug test. Will you take it now?"

I told my clients that I had to drive to a lab and take a hair follicle test, which would determine whether I had used drugs—within the last six months.

"If I had smoked marijuana while I was out of work, even six months before I was even looking for the job, or had any concept that I would have the opportunity to work at this great job, I would have been immediately excluded from consideration!" I would say.

I thought about my brother, Bert, at times like this, and how he had lost his job after a failed drug test. For all that I learned in my work as a substance abuse counselor, and for all the inspiration I felt in helping people find recovery, my destiny was not to continue in the Quest program.

Opportunity knocked. I had the chance to become an outpatient therapist at DMCC. My own therapists in Huntsville, Marilyn and later Bernice, worked in the outpatient program there, and becoming an outpatient therapist was my ultimate goal. It was impossible not to answer this new challenge. I experienced so many changes in my life through the years, and I continued to "roll with the flow" of them, as they presented themselves to me.

TO ANOTHER SHORE

In the early months of winter 2006, the program director of the DMCC, Mike, the man who had given me my start as a therapist, announced he was retiring. A man named Scott would be taking his position as the program director. This shift left a vacancy in the outpatient program. I did not particularly want to leave the Quest program so quickly, and felt that I had much more to learn about treating people with addiction.

I felt obligated to myself, though, to apply for the job opening, since it had been my long-standing dream. I didn't know when, if ever, this opportunity might appear again. Therefore, with a heavy heart, I told my friends, colleagues, and clients at Quest of my decision.

Within two weeks, I began my new job as an outpatient therapist, pleased that I had met my goal in just two years of full-time employment. Mike told me, laughingly, that I didn't know what I was getting into, and he was certainly correct. This new position proved even more demanding than the other positions I had worked in at MHCNCA.

I had to completely readjust my concept of time, because I was scheduled to see people either individually or in a group session for eight hours each day. This meant that if I had matters I needed to take care of in my personal life during work hours, I had to plan for them about a month in advance.

I also had to learn the process of the complicated scheduling system, and how all of this related to the computer system we had online at the MHCNA.

This was all entirely new to me, since at my other positions I had scheduled individual appointments on an as-needed basis. Because of these demands on my time, I was compelled to cancel my status as a client at the HMCMHC. I simply didn't think I could continue to manage the long drive to Huntsville and back to keep my appointments with my therapist and psychiatrist there while meeting the requirements of my own clients.

The HMCMHC had saved my life, and had been available when I needed it most. It was very difficult for me to stop attending appointments there. What I did not know at the time, though, was that my affiliation there was far from over, in ways I could not have predicted.

I dedicated myself to mastering all the skills I needed to provide quality therapeutic service as an outpatient therapist. I had done extensive work with people with psychotic disorders, depression, and substance abuse disorders throughout my career. I was surprised when I realized that in my new position, there was a disorder about which I knew nothing. Many of my new clients were suffering from panic disorder or other forms of anxiety disorder, which I had never treated in my two years of working as a therapist. And I had not had any extensive discussion with people who lived with these disorders in all my professional contacts with mentally ill clients.

I was not intimidated, however, and began researching the topic of how to treat people with anxiety disorders. Within a week's time, I was completely familiar with all the latest research on how to treat people therapeutically with this disorder. Like other SMI, medication was an important part of treatment, and I learned more about Xanax, Klonopin, and other benzodiazepines, which are beneficial to people in recovery from these disorders.

Another new aspect to this position was that I was now responsible for assessing people new to DMCC, and filling out all of the documentation necessary for them to be clients.

I would give a diagnostic impression of what mental illness I thought the person had, and what types of services they would be eligible to receive. The psychiatrist would later render the actual diagnosis after reading my diagnostic impression and interviewing the client. People would often come tearfully to me, in a state of hopelessness. It was my job to fill out the complicated set of forms, and determine what set of diagnostic criteria they met, if any.

During these moments, I would think back to the time when I was assessed at the HMCMHC, literally at the brink of suicide. I thought back to how cold and austere the person who assessed me seemed; although now I understood exactly why it had to be that way. I had the responsibility to do an accurate assessment, leaving no question unanswered, in a very limited amount of time.

I did everything I could in these situations to avoid this sense of cold detachment. At times, it was very difficult to keep the necessary distance. The best technique I learned was taught to me by, Sharon, another therapist in the outpatient program.

She reminded me very much of the therapists who had worked with me over the years. I had great respect for her. She said I should make a disclaimer to the client at the beginning of the assessment, telling him or her that I would not have an opportunity to do any real therapy at the initial session, and that I did not mean to seem impersonal, though I might appear to be.

This admonition often fell upon deaf ears though, and I found myself providing a great deal of comfort and encouragement to these people during the assessment phase, whether I had the time or not. What I discovered was that despite my best efforts at managing time, there never really seemed to be enough time to do all of the things expected of me.

I worked as an outpatient therapist for about ten months, increasing my mastery of time management, when a position in Day Treatment, the job I had worked in when I first began at the MHCNCA, opened. There were a great many characteristics to that position that I preferred to the outpatient program position, which had proven very unlike what I had expected. Therefore, in March 2007, I accepted a transfer back to the Day Treatment program.

It didn't take a long time back in the Day Treatment program to validate my decision to move back there. In the outpatient program, there was almost no opportunity to have discussions with other staff within the program.

There had been barely enough time to have a session with a client and then work on the endless paperwork involved before seeing the next client. The clients in the outpatient program were mostly those who were higher functioning than the clients in Day Treatment. Crisis situations where more than one staff member were required to handle a situation were rare.

Day treatment, by contrast, was a team effort, where constant communication with other staff was vital. In Day Treatment, crises occurred on an if not daily, then certainly weekly basis. A client might be having a medical complaint, a conflict with another client, or might be feeling suicidal. While this facet of providing treatment may have proved daunting to many clinicians, for me, managing crisis-situations had practically become second nature. My ability to handle crises had been strengthened by the fact that I had lived such a tumultuous life.

The other staff knew me for my ability to remain exceptionally calm under pressure. In my previous job in the outpatient program, I was called upon to handle crisis situations when they arose. My reputation for staying unruffled grew when I returned to Day Treatment, and I quickly fit in with the staff, though they were all new to me.

The clients who were still in Day Treatment, saddened by my earlier departure, welcomed me back with open arms. I brought back with me all of the knowledge which I had acquired in my work with Quest and the outpatient program. I spoke to the Day Treatment clients as a group, assuring them that I would use all the knowledge I had acquired in my work with these other programs for their betterment. My goal was to improve their lives, and I would do everything in my power to make sure they received the quality of care they deserved.

In March of 2007, I earned my license as a certified social worker. This gave me a substantial increase in pay and the ability to provide services for additional people whose insurance required that they be treated by a person with my license.

At this point in my life, the idea to set the events of my life in writing began to become more insistent. I remembered the words of the law professor who told me, "Write a book," when speaking to me after the submission of my application to law school. Coworkers began encouraging me to tell my story. They told me that my accomplishments could be an inspiration to other people.

It was now April of 2007, and there was a movie out on DVD that captured my attention, called Stranger than Fiction, starring Will Farrell. In the movie, the main character was living his life, only to discover that he was a character in a book written by another person. I felt I could relate to the character in the movie. My life had become more than just the fulfillment of my own goals and desires. It was an open book, which would inspire other people if they knew my story. This meant that every important decision I made, or any momentous occasion I experienced, would be recorded by my own hand. This was a surreal sensation. I found it tough to become accustomed to the fact that I lived a life that would be examined by many. I continued my work, without pause.

AMAZEMENT

I telephoned my old therapist, Bernice, after about eleven months of having not spoken to her, letting her know I had obtained my license as a certified social worker. She congratulated me, telling me how proud she was of what I had accomplished. She also said that she would be leaving the HMCMHC, as she was taking on a position in another town. We said our farewells and I thought that it would be some time until I had the chance to speak with her again.

To my surprise, I received a call from Bernice a couple of weeks later. She had a question: she asked if I would be willing to accept an award from the HMCMHC, at its annual luncheon. As a former member of the Consumer Council, I had attended several of these luncheons over the years, and I knew that they were comprised of about one hundred people who worked for the HMCMHC, members of the Consumer Council, and many other officials within the city of Huntsville and Madison County.

I happily told Bernice that I would certainly accept an award if it was offered. She called again a couple of days later, informing me that I had been chosen to receive the award. The prize I was accepting was the first annual Beacon of Hope Award, which would recognize a Consumer of Mental Health Services for the inspiration he provided to others.

The new director of the HMCMHC, Brian Davis, and the clinical director, Anne Murray, made the final selection to honor me with this award. While I was certainly grateful to be selected out of all the many thousands of clients from the HMCMHC, many of whom had gone on to accomplish extraordinary feats in their own right, there was a part of me that had misgivings about accepting the award.

It had become ingrained in me to try to hide the fact that I had a mental illness from almost everyone that I knew. It was now difficult for me to be seen as a PLMI, especially in front of such a large number of people. I had spent years honing my skills as a social worker, and craved recognition for being a quality therapist in my own right, without the qualification of being in recovery from schizophrenia.

I spoke about these reservations with my new supervisor, in whom I had confided the facts about my mental illness. I felt comfortable talking with him about these matters. He helped allay any misgivings I had about the award by helping me to see that an opportunity to accept an award in our field was "few and far between," so I prepared myself for this honor the best way I knew how.

Accepting the award meant that I had to drive to the HMCMHC and be interviewed on video, which would later be edited for presentation at the luncheon. This was an ingenious idea, in that it spared the recipient from the stress of having to prepare a speech and deliver it in front of a large crowd.

I was delighted to meet with Brian Davis and Anne Murray in one of the offices at the HMCMHC. I answered a series of necessarily personal questions, in front of a camera, about my past struggle with serious mental illness.

While on video, I spoke at length about how the mental health center was the only place I had to turn to for support, and how it had been like a family to me over the past decade. I talked about the experience of being diagnosed with schizophrenia, and of how much it had altered and shaped my adult life. I described how I had lost many of the people who were closest to me in my life, and how I was introduced to an entirely new group of people, who through my experiences had become very important to me.

Before I was to receive my award, though, I was to participate in another grand event. It was a conference of the Community Mental Health Centers from throughout the state, which met in Birmingham. This conference was attended not only by the professionals who I had worked with for years in Decatur, but also by professionals who had worked with me for years in Huntsville.

This experience was a further test of my ability to walk the tight rope of sharing an experience with people who knew about my history of mental illness, and others who did not.

I attended a lecture held by Marilyn, my first therapist at the HMCMHC, about how to work with people suffering from grief and loss. This was an extraordinary experience for me, as I am sure it was for Marilyn. I had only seen her once or twice in the last seven years. She had, however, been such an important lifeline throughout the first five years after my initial diagnosis. Now I was attending the same conference at which she was speaking; it was ironic that I was attending as an experienced mental health professional.

My attendance at this conference was a pivotal point in my life for many reasons, but one of the most important was that I met a unique man, Walter Ballard. He would prove to be a force for change in my life as great as any other individual.

Walter had recently been hired to a management position at the HMCMHC and had worked in a wide array of helping professions since his retirement from the military. He was a black man in his fifties, with a wiry frame. His compassionate spirit shone through, and we had an instant connection.

I confided in Walter about the award I would be receiving, since I would be seeing him at the luncheon in a couple of days. When he asked me if I was interested in spreading the news of my personal story, I informed him that I was.

Walter handed me his business card and asked me to attend the presentation he was giving the next day. I went to hear him give a presentation on the Medicaid and Medicare health insurance programs, in which he had become an expert. Walter had brought three different projectors for his presentation, and when all of them failed to function properly, he handed everyone paper copies of his presentation, which he had made just in case. I found this level of foresight quite impressive. I was equally dazzled with the way Walter was able to make an otherwise dry topic interesting, through his ability to communicate effectively with his audience.

Little did I know at that time how important a friend and mentor Walter would become. Nor did I know how much his influence would shape my life for the better. Walter had the ability to inspire people, and he utilized this ability to motivate me to strive for excellence.

When I attended an award luncheon held at the conference, I was surprised to see that Marie Hood, the Executive Director for the Mental Health Center of North Central Alabama, was the chairperson for the entire statewide body who had put the conference together.

I realized that Marie was the head official for the mental health systems of three counties, what I did not realize was that she was an official of great import for the entire state of Alabama. Later on, at what would be considered a festive dinner, Mrs. Hood approached me and told me that she had spoken to Brian Davis, the Executive Director of the HMCMHC, about my upcoming award.

"I told Brian that you were a good choice," she confided.

This made me feel more confident about the situation, and I deeply appreciated her support. My head began to swim at this dinner as the confluence of two great forces in my life came together. They were in the form of the staff at the HMCMHC, who had played such a tremendous role in my life, and the staff at the MHCNCA, including Mrs. Hood, who was an integral part of my life as well.

After the conference, I drove back to Decatur both tired and excited by all I had experienced. I rested and prepared myself as much as I could for the award luncheon at which I was to accept the Beacon of Hope Award. Shortly before the luncheon, I was briefed by Brian Davis about what to expect, and I saw the edited video of my interview.

Seeing myself on video was a unique experience, for which I was little prepared. I had mannerisms that seemed somewhat at odds with the way I had always pictured myself. Viewing my profile, I thought I could see a certain flat expression that I recognized in my clients. They had similar disorders to mine, although I had never noticed this lack of emotions in my own facial expressions. I found it very difficult to watch myself on the screen.

Another characteristic that I noticed when watching myself on the tiny screen, was the horror-stricken look in my eyes as I described the events of my life in detail. It was clear, that the person in this tape might still be struggling to come to terms with the diagnosis that had shaped his life so fundamentally. He seemed to be in a state of shock about what had happened to him ten years ago.

The person I was seeing was utterly transformed by his experiences. The fact was written clearly on his face, as he described it. The closing discussion of the tape showed the person describing great strides he had made, and how he had managed to put his life in order. Somehow that distant look of wonder and confusion about what had happened never seemed to completely leave his face. The person in the video seemed to have as many questions remaining as he did answers, although he was determined to live his life to the fullest extent possible.

Grateful for the fact that I had been prepared, to some extent, for what was to come next, Eleanor and I made the trip to Huntsville for the award luncheon. We sat at a table with the members of the Consumer Council, whom I had known for many years. Another person who sat with us was my friend Tim Jennings-Carr. I have heard it said, and I believe it, that the difference between someone having a successful recovery or not could be greatly determined by whether or not the person in question has one friend in his life. In my case, Tim had been my one friend in many of the darkest times in my recovery when I had no other friends. He had been friends with David and Bill, the two men in the story who were my adopted siblings throughout my childhood. He was tall with long black hair, and he had played drums in a variety of bands throughout his life. He was also gifted with the ability to repair literally everything. When I was a freshman in college at UA, he was a senior. We ran into one another there and spent a lot of time together that year. While I worked as a security officer at the mall, he ran into me there and we renewed our friendship. We watched many Alabama Crimson Tide football games on television together, and listening to his bands play always helped to improve my mood.

Many people received awards that day, and there were numerous speeches made by public officials and clergy.

At the climax of the luncheon, the edited video was projected on a large screen in front of the one-hundred or so people. While I had been prepared for what to expect in the video, what I was not prepared for was the reaction of the audience.

People were weeping quite audibly about what they saw on the screen, and it was clear to everyone present that the moment was an exceptionally moving one. Brian asked if I would like to get up and say a few words. As I made my way to the lectern in the center of a line of officials sitting perpendicular to the audience, I cleared my throat, preparing to speak. My initial instinct to say something humorous I could now see was a good one, since the sheer solemnity of the occasion seemed almost palpable.

"Well, this is the first time I've ever been asked to follow myself before, but here goes!" I said.

The tension lifted a bit by the crowd's reaction to my humor. I now found myself able to actually look at the mass of faces gazing expectantly at me.

I thanked God for allowing me to receive the award, and then all of the people I could recall who had helped. I tried to go on speaking some of the haphazard lines which had formed in my mind, but found myself unable to do so as my nervousness essentially caused me to freeze up.

It felt very much like my brain had locked in place somehow, as I realized that whatever characteristics about my own expressions I thought I saw on the screen, must certainly be in full bloom at this moment. My initial success at lightening the mood of the crowd and remembering to thank most of the people I should have stood in stark contrast to the sense of paralysis I now felt as I fumbled for something to say.

Matters became worse because of my sense of self-consciousness about having schizophrenia, and my fear that my inability to articulate what I wanted to say would be seen as associated somehow with my mental illness. The mood grew grave once more, as my sense of being overwhelmed must have become obvious to the crowd.

Ironically, when working with much smaller groups of people in a group therapy setting, I felt much more comfortable and certainly did not exhibit this same sense of unease.

I left the podium to applause, award in hand, to take my place back with the people at my table. I was truly thankful to be the recipient of the award, but left the luncheon thinking much the way I did after the speech I'd made when we started Our Place. I realized that I should become much better at public speaking before trying again.

I returned to work in Decatur, placing my award atop the cabinet in my office. I realized how fortunate I was to have received my award. Most professionals who practice in community mental health work daily for little pay and practically no recognition for the immense service they provide in touching other people's lives. I now saw with fresh eyes just how special a group of people they really are. They work unceasingly to improve the lives of their fellow men and women, without any expectations of fortune or fame.

The concept of writing a book to share more widely the story of overcoming mental illness was constantly in my thoughts. I yearned to find guidance for this project. I decided to call Walter Ballard to seek whatever counsel he was willing to provide.

When I telephoned him, I found him very receptive to my goals, and I discovered that he was very knowledgeable about the avenues I must take to spread my message of hope. After our first long telephone conversation, I emailed him the early draft of my manuscript, which, at the time consisted of approximately thirty pages of text. Walter telephoned me back in a few days and began in earnest to shape my life in ways I could not yet comprehend. He helped me to see that writing was only a part of the larger picture of what I must become to see my life and work transform the lives of others.

He helped me to see that I must become a master communicator, proficient not only in writing but in public speaking. I felt very comfortable in speaking to groups of people in therapy sessions I facilitated, since I had years of experience in the process. But providing group therapy is a much different animal from successfully delivering a public speech.

Group therapy is about listening to other people and expanding on their ideas, as much as anything. In a public speech, there is one speaker and it is incumbent upon him to provide all of the necessary information to his audience, in a concise, clear, and entertaining way.

Walter convinced me that I must now become as familiar with the discipline of public speaking as I was with any of my other skills. He then began to show me his true genius as a motivator. Walter, in essence, became my life coach, and spoke to me for hours on the telephone, helping to bring out the potential that he saw in me. He told me that I might want to check out an organization designed to improve public speakers: the Toastmasters. I found the nearest Toastmaster's meeting on the internet and immediately joined.

The next thing that Walter did was to convince me to read motivational books. Reading books such as John Maxwell's, *Talent is Never Enough*, it became clear to me that I was not living up to my full potential. The essential messages of these books was that one can attain his or her ambitions by setting clear goals and then making all of the effort required to see them become a reality. My life and the accomplishments I had made thus far were certainly testament to this truth, as I resolved to do all that was required to see my next dream become a reality.

My new dream was to complete the writing of a book which would inspire others, and to make its message available to everyone who would benefit from it. This meant that I had to learn to work on it consistently in order to create the contents of my message, while at the same time balancing all of the demands from work, family, and my newfound desire to master public speaking. Walter believed in me, and in my message of hope, and he understood its power to effect positive change, as well as to touch lives throughout the world. His belief was a great catalyst for transforming me into a person on a crusade to better the lives of others on a vast scale, and into a man who was rapidly developing the tools necessary for making this dream a reality.

Another concept that Walter worked diligently to drum into my mind was that I must become a master of time. Time management was the key element in my quest to see my vision become a reality. Walter explained that a physician was able to survive the rigors of medical school and attain his professional status because he was able to master the dimension of time.

Time not spent on productive activity had to be considered and factored against all of the time available. I could accomplish major undertakings simply by deciding how much time to set aside for a specific activity and then living up to the plan. In writing my book, for example, I would have to decide what amount of time that I could spare every week in writing. Walter did not care one whit about how long it took to arrive at a finished product, as long as I was working on it consistently and reaching the goals I had set for myself.

Walter Ballard taught me these concepts and much more. He had prepared answers to just about any problem that I could pose for him related to my life and goals, and he was there to discuss anything that might be on my mind. He had become a true mentor, and a friend.

Walter was working on a book on excellence and had mastered the art of public speaking. His sheer genius for motivation is something that transformed my life. Spreading my message of hope had now become a solid commitment.

WORLDS COLLIDE

One feature of my new sense of motivation was that I felt like a more magnetic person. My thought that I would one day go on to deliver a powerful message to a receptive audience was on the forefront of my consciousness. Indeed, one of the primary ways that I learned to make this goal happen was to visualize it regularly, and to actively think about the result and ways in which I would ensure its success.

Without being able to visualize the end result, goals of great import to the rest of the world are nearly impossible. I believed in myself and in my goals; that's what really mattered most. A byproduct of all of this, I discovered, was that other people could see this change in me, as well. My new sense of self-confidence was clear to anyone who spent any length of time with me, and I sensed that other people believed in me! It took some time for me to become accustomed to my new realization of life and its possibilities.

Luckily, though, time was something I had in abundance. I realized that my dreams would not come into fruition overnight, and that the only way they would become a reality was through the steady application of the techniques I had learned over time. All other goals I had accomplished had required the same elements of consistent work, and I just had to apply myself in a similar fashion, although on a much grander scale. I was becoming a more rounded person in many ways through my efforts, and I was gaining an increased ability to establish rapport with other people, including some of the people who meant the most to me—my clients.

In May 2007, Eleanor and I had been married for a year and a half. She and I were visiting her parents at their new house, on the ritzy side of Decatur. I was in the middle of regaling them with my newfound sense of purpose that I was putting into positive action. I was talking about the new speeches I was writing and committing to memory for Toastmasters, and of the now steady progress I was making toward completing my book.

In the middle of explaining all the projects I was working on, my mother-in-law began questioning me about my brother Bert. She often asked about my childhood and my past, and I often had difficulty explaining it to her, since my life had been so profoundly different from most other people.

I explained to her the difficulty I had encountered in trying to help Bert and attempted to describe to her how unreceptive he had been to mental health treatment. I found that the powerful resistance I had experienced in trying to help Bert was something difficult for me to frame into words. I failed in my efforts to convince my in-laws that there was nothing more that I could do to help Bert, and the questions they were putting to me rang in my ears with the implication that I should be doing more.

"Well, he is part of your family, after all," my mother-in-law, said.

"It might be a good idea for you to at least try and talk to him," my father-in-law pointed out.

I think the factor that most alarmed them about the situation was that I had absolutely no knowledge of where my brother was, or how he was faring.

"He might have been hit by a car or something," my father-in-law suggested.

I told them I felt certain in my heart that nothing of that severity had befallen Bert. Remembering well Bert's seemingly limitless penchant for survival, I told them, "It would take an atom bomb!" For that was the dilemma inherent in any prior attempts to assist Bert.

Bert could be in a psychotic state for a very long time without breaking down completely.

He could toil away in a stressful work environment, the whole while experiencing severe psychotic symptoms. He could live with the symptoms long enough to maintain employment at the same job for a year or so. Then when he began responding to his symptoms by yelling at them in an uncontrollable fashion, he would be asked by his employer to leave.

Bert would invariably find support at the missions, whenever his inability to function independently came to the fore. Bert didn't accept that he had mental illness despite clear evidence to the contrary.

When he did live at the mission, the staff there was constantly trying to convince him to take his medication. They would force him to keep appointments at the HMCMHC, to enforce taking his medication. Obviously, they found his psychotic symptoms to be as difficult to live with as his employers did, and as I had.

Bert experienced symptoms to a greater degree and for a much longer period than did many others in his condition who, much sooner than Bert, accepted assistance from the mental health community.

I was not able to explain Bert and his problems to Eleanor's parents, and they soon convinced me that me not knowing the actual whereabouts or condition of my brother and his status was wrong, and constituted a situation that I should make efforts to modify.

"Don't you think your grandmother would want you to make an effort to contact Bert, and make sure he's okay?" my mother-in-law asked.

At this point in the conversation, my ire was truly sparked.

"I may not be a saint, but my grandmother was, as sure as anyone! Of course she would want me to go find him!" I proclaimed.

I promised Eleanor's mother that I would go and seek Bert within the next couple of days. I would at least try to determine where he lived and his current condition.

When Eleanor and I left their home, I felt that no one in the family understood the full ramifications of what they were asking of me. I hoped that the years of training that I now had as a mental health therapist would bolster my ability to face this new challenge.

The trepidation I experienced about having to try to deal with Bert's situation was at odds with the concern that I had for him as my brother. I had tried as much as I could to block out my own worry for his well-being. He had not wanted my help up to this point and I had not thought of myself as in a position to provide him the help he needed. Despite the mental barriers I had erected, I often found my mind wandering to my brother's welfare. These thoughts had a greater tendency to arise during the holidays when I would think about what Bert might be doing, and how he must feel to be alone. During the nights before I made my trip to search for Bert, these thoughts that had been bottled up inside my subconscious overflowed into my conscious mind and became a burning drive to make contact with him, despite my unease about the situation.

In preparing myself mentally to find Bert, I thought about how most of the times I had spoken to him in the last ten years, he was in a state of psychosis. His mental state made it extremely difficult to communicate with him or to convince him of anything. I thought that when I did find him he would be in a similar state, and I didn't know what I would do next. I knew I could not have him admitted to the hospital unless he proved a danger to himself or others, a concept which had always been so difficult to prove, in Bert's case. I did my best to prepare myself for seeing Bert in that condition. Observing Bert's psychosis always opened a floodgate of emotions.

On the Sunday morning following my discussion with Eleanor's parents, I went to Huntsville to answer the calling I now felt: to find Bert. The last time I had spoken to him on the phone nearly two years ago, and he had been living and working at a plant in Madison, a large suburb of Huntsville. I figured there was more than a sixty percent chance that he had relapsed by that time, and was now back at the mission in Huntsville, where he frequently stayed. In any event, the mission was the only place I knew to look for him, thinking that they might at least know in which direction to point me if he was not living there.

I arrived at the Breaking Free Rescue Mission, located just two blocks from the Shelter Plus apartment complex I had lived in for seven years. The monastic feel that pervaded the interior of the mission was still there. A darkened auditorium filled with pews was clearly visible upon entering. People who live at the mission are a particularly spiritual lot, by necessity. They are required to attend religious services daily.

Bert was the most spiritual person I had ever encountered, assuming stubbornness was not counted as a sin, and I could understand why he felt a sense of solace there.

There was an office off to the side, which was just as dark as the rest of the interior. I approached a man standing in the office doorway. He was wearing dark sunglasses, and was otherwise modestly dressed in a threadbare shirt and blue jeans. The "no frills" short-sleeved, collared shirt and slacks I was wearing seemed an ostentatious extravagance in this place of simplicity. He said that Bert had left the mission just two days before. After he'd been living at the mission for the past six months, he'd suddenly moved out. We both knew that the best place to search for Bert next was at one of the other rescue missions.

With a hope and a prayer, I traveled the five miles or so to the Downtown Rescue Mission to find if my brother had moved there. I parked my car at the mission, thinking of the time or two I had eaten a free meal there, wondering what it must be like to live there for an extended time. When I asked for Bert at the front desk station, the two men there said that they didn't know him.

An African American man, dressed much like me, approached me, asking for a description of Bert.

"Is he tall?" he asked.

"Yes, he is," I replied.

He then led me to a place that made quite an impact upon me and will no doubt haunt my thoughts for the rest of my life.

We went to a large building away from the main area. On a large concrete floor, about twenty scantily clad men lay sleeping in a large circle. Most of them were using a t-shirt or other bits of cloth for a pillow. After overcoming the initial shock of seeing such a gruesome spectacle, one of the men came into clearer focus; it was Bert!

"That's him!" I said.

The kindly gentleman who'd led me to the place went away.

It was Bert lying on the ground, with only a t-shirt to cushion him from the cold, hard, seamless concrete floor. The floodgate of emotions rose in me much quicker than I had anticipated, as I sat cross-legged next to Bert's sleeping form and woke him.

He overcame his initial surprise of seeing me as I focused on keeping the emotions churned up by the situation from overwhelming me.

"Oh, hey man," he said, in that voice that everyone said sounded so much like my own.

One thing I was struck by, after a few exchanges with him, was that Bert was not in the psychotic state I had expected. He was clear eyed and responding appropriately to everything I asked him.

"Do you want to go for a drive with me?" I asked.

"Sure, man," he replied.

I soon determined that the reason Bert was not in a psychotic state was that the Breaking Free Rescue Mission, where he had been living for the last six months, had been requiring him to take his medication, and had been making him stay free from substance abuse.

Bert had been working at the local family restaurant where he had worked on and off for years washing dishes. He said that he had become overwhelmed by the stress of the job and with one of the people working in the kitchen. This prompted him to leave the Breaking Free Rescue Mission to come to the Down Town Rescue Mission. "I've only been off my medication for a couple of days," he said.

Bert was surprised that I had become a therapist and now had a wife and a house in Decatur. He had been in a state of psychosis earlier times when I told him I was a therapist. I suppose my explanations at that time just did not register. It turned out that he had even been in a state of psychosis when he spoke to me on the telephone two years ago. At that time, he had been considering giving me his car, not understanding that I had completely transformed my life.

Shortly after the telephone call two years ago, Bert's psychotic symptoms led to the police being called to his job site. The result was that Bert was dragged off, not to return. Bert had two bags of marijuana on him at the time. He was ordered to pay heavy fines by the court, although he received no jail time. The judge ordered Bert to attend New Horizons. New Horizons was the Substance Abuse Outpatient Program in Huntsville, which was part of the Mental Health Center, similar to Quest, the program in which I had been a counselor in Decatur.

Bert had sold his car to pay the fines, and soon found himself back at the mission and his job at the restaurant, since he was the only one in the mission who really didn't mind working there.

I was now having a rational conversation in my car with Bert for the first time in six years. The feeling was surreal as I drove Bert to Cheeburger Cheeburger to have lunch, reveling in my ability to communicate with a man who, finally, was coherent.

I promised Bert I would try to help him get on his feet. I began trying to convince him to return to the Breaking Free Rescue Mission, where they had been requiring him to take his medication, saying that I would speak to the people at the HMCMHC and ask them to allow him return to the housing program where they had once granted him admittance, or to some other program.

I told Bert that I would help him apply for disability income, for which he had been denied. The program at the Mental Health Center, which helped Bert to receive his medication at a reduced cost, had mandated that Bert at least apply for disability insurance the previous year. Bert had not been eligible at that time since he was working full time.

After several hours, I drove back to Decatur, alone, with Bert's assurance that he would return to the Breaking Free Rescue Mission. I was determined to help him gain access to the full package of benefits for which he was eligible. The drive, however, left me feeling unfulfilled. I returned to my house feeling a mixture of thankfulness that I had found Bert and frustration that he was still homeless.

At home, I told Eleanor all that I had experienced and soon found myself so overcome with emotion that I began weeping onto our pillows. Lying in our bed together, she asked me what I wanted to do.

I said, "Let's just go get him."

I was resigned in my heart to do what some part of me knew we must do.

When we made the drive back to Huntsville together it was late afternoon, and we saw a most beautiful sight. Hot air balloons, one of the things for which Decatur is renowned, were making their Memorial Day flights, and the low hanging sun shone a dusky orange on their colorful silks. All manner of balloons were taking off to journey to wherever it is these lofty vehicles ascend in their fantastical flights.

After a few minutes, the balloons were behind us as we journeyed into the unknown depths of our own lives. I knew how many people had allowed Bert to move in with them in the past, and I shuddered to think about how unprepared they must have been whenever Bert had reached a state where he could no longer stay with them. I was now a veteran in working with PLMI, and I realized that I would have my work cut out for me meeting this new challenge. I was on my way now to face a reality, which had been, for years, the theme of a recurring nightmare.

The nightmare was one in which Bert had somehow moved back in with me, displacing me from my home. It persisted, fresh in my mind, though I had screwed up my courage to face my darkest fears. Mine was a mindset completely different from my wife's, who had never experienced the constant barrage of incoherent speech that is part of living with someone who is actively psychotic. In her mind, someone in my family was in need, and we were going to help him, because that was what one's family must do.

When we arrived at the mission to announce the good news to Bert, we found that he had moved on once more to the Salvation Army Mission. I realized then that my instinct to move Bert in the house with us was the right one, since I thought it doubtful that he would return to the Breaking Free Rescue Mission where they made him take his medicine.

It was dusk, and we had some difficulty finding the mission. It was located in a housing project area, where Eleanor had never been; but it was familiar to me. I had surveyed that area for the Census Bureau, years before. We walked to the front desk and asked for Bert. We were told that he was among the residents currently attending religious services, but that they should be returning in a van any minute now.

There we waited in our car for Bert to return, surrounded by some residents who were conversing outside. Apparently they had chosen not to go to the religious service.

Bert returned in the van, as promised. Eleanor and I immediately began talking him into coming to live with us, for as long as it took for him to get a home of his own. We drove back to Decatur feeling a sense of relief, and the powerful sense of euphoria one experiences when doing something that will profoundly, and positively, affect the life of another.

My grandmother had asked me a long time ago to do everything in my power to help my brother, and now I was not only in a position to do that, but I was fulfilling her wishes as promised.

I had thought Grandmother overly optimistic when she had charged me with this responsibility so many years ago. I could not envision myself in any real position to take on such a difficult challenge. Now I could see the foresight intrinsic in her request.

As amazing a feeling as it was to be a benefit to my own family, I found myself thinking about the other men who were lying on that concrete floor with Bert. These men didn't have a brother who had gained vast knowledge about mental health and how to help people with mental illnesses. They didn't have a family member who was a social worker and who was willing to take on the challenge of awakening them so that they might enter a new world. Indeed, it was highly unlikely that a person who has surpassed great odds would reappear in their lives to help them create a storybook ending.

I really didn't think that most people in our society realized that one can walk into a mission in one of the world's most prosperous cities, on any given day, and witness a sight as horrific as I'd beheld: twenty men lying inertly on a concrete floor as if they had lost all hope in living. I had never imagined such a scene, and I had worked with the most marginalized segment of the population for years.

AN ODD TRIO

Bert moved into an incredibly shrinking house with Eleanor and me. I soon discovered that the difficulty I had in interacting with my brother didn't apply to Eleanor and her family, who seemed to get along better with Bert, in many instances, than they did with me. Bert and Eleanor enjoyed watching movies together while I would write, read, and engage in other solitary pursuits.

Eleanor and her family appreciated Bert's reappearance in my life because before this, they had seen me as someone largely without a family or any reminder of my past. Bert was the embodiment of my roots, and they welcomed him with open arms. My own interactions with Bert were more problematic.

One reason my relationship with Bert was awkward for me had to do with the past. Bert was now entirely free of psychotic symptoms and was very similar to the people Eleanor and I had both worked with over the years, who were now coping successfully with their symptoms.

My view of Bert went deeper though. I recalled the difficulty I had experienced while Bert was in the full throes of psychosis. The second, and final, severe psychotic break that I experienced happened when Bert and I were living with Grandmother. It was attributable in no small measure to the constant presence of the symptoms Bert was experiencing.

Before either Bert or I had ever exhibited any psychotic symptoms, we were constantly at odds with one another. Our relationship had evolved from Bert as a constant tormentor, to Bert as a potential rival for my grandmother's affection and a violator of my personal space.

After Bert developed mental illness, he experienced a pervasive guilt about bullying me during childhood.

"That's all water under the bridge, Bert. I don't even think about that stuff anymore," I would tell him.

"I just can't get it out of my head," was his reply.

My relationship with Bert was also made difficult by the fact that I saw in Bert many of my own foibles that I found disturbing. His mental illness, mannerisms, and personality were so similar to mine; he was like a constant reminder in my home of the things that made me feel self-conscious.

While Bert was living with us, I took advantage of the fact that he was knowledgeable about several technical matters. Bert and I journeyed to the local Wal-Mart to buy stereo equipment to enhance our home entertainment center. Before Bert had his first psychotic break, he had earned good money at plant jobs, and had spent much of it on high-value stereo equipment. He was now truly amazed at the prices of the electronics at the store. It was as if he had missed the trend of electronics going down in price altogether while in the throes of his illness; like Rip Van Winkle, he had been out of touch with the society around him.

While at Wal-Mart, I also researched and determined the best deal on cell phones. I bought Bert a phone, and was surprised to learn I could purchase a phone with a plan that would meet his needs for eighteen dollars down and thirty dollars every two months. He was completely unfamiliar with cell phones, as he was with so much in this new electronic age, and had been making calls on pay phones. Stereo equipment, though, was virtually unchanged, except for price, and he was able to accomplish something that I couldn't. He installed our new home surround sound system.

In my efforts to find Bert a home of his own, I soon found myself in a quandary. Bert was now living in Decatur with us, but he had lived in Huntsville for most of his life. It seemed like a conflict of interest to try to help Bert receive mental health services through my employer. Although, since he was now a Decatur resident, I could see how it could possibly be the only place for him to turn. Bert was already a client at the HMCMHC, and had been attending a group therapy session there once every three months. I thought the best thing to do was to contact his therapist for a family session.

Bert's therapist, Mary Beth, spoke kindly on the telephone and scheduled a time for us to meet with her. When we met, I realized I had actually spoken with Mary Beth before at the Mental Health Center. When I was in a psychotic state, shortly before being committed to NARH, she had been the therapist that spoke with me in my state of crisis while my own therapist was out of the office. I also had a memorable, but silent, encounter with her when we shared an elevator at the hospital during the time leading up to my grandmother's passing.

Mary Beth said that since he was only living with me temporarily, he could continue to receive services at the HMCMHC. She also said that she would refer Bert to case management in order to assist him in finding a place to live.

I took Bert to the SSA office in Decatur to apply for Social Security disability benefits. Bert needed to produce a birth certificate; he had been born in New Orleans, Louisiana, which had been devastated by hurricane Katrina two years earlier, and we had no idea if his birth certificate still existed. I was later able to order Bert's birth certificate over the internet, with no problem. The archives containing the record of his birth had survived the flood.

The major problem was finding him housing before he began receiving disability payments, since our best estimate was that it might take Bert an entire year to win his disability case. In my experience, that seemed about the average time a person had to wait. I have known people who waited five years to receive disability payments. The prospect of having Bert live with us for an entire year was not one I savored, although I was willing to endure it in order to see him off the street.

I telephoned Bert's case manager to ask him about the possibility of Bert finding a place in the Shelter Plus Program, where I had lived for seven years. I knew from personal experience that one could live there for a time without steady income. Bert's case manager didn't sound particularly encouraging about Bert's prospects for receiving a placement in the program, so I settled in for a long wait.

Bert did not believe in his heart that he would be eligible for Social Security disability payments. To him it sounded too good to be true, especially in light of the fact that he had already been turned down for Social Security Disability Income.

His hopelessness was in spite of my constant assurances that he was not only now eligible, but also that he had greater symptomatic problems than many of the people I had worked with over the years who were receiving disability payments.

Matters became worse when the attorney who had helped with my disability case, and who I now retained to help Bert, seemed discouraged because Bert had done so much work in the recent past. I constantly encouraged Bert, in every way I could, as the days of our living together turned into months.

During this time, I continued to make progress in public speaking, enjoying the personal growth I was developing through Toastmasters. One of the members of the group, Marilyn Volanino, was someone I had already come to know, since she was the President of the National Alliance on Mental Illness in Decatur.

Walter continued to hammer into my brain the principles of diligence and consistent effort. I continued to make progress in writing and speaking and was becoming what Walter termed a "Master Communicator." I traveled to Huntsville on several occasions to watch Walter give a series of speeches on financial matters to a group of people from the community. After the presentation, Walter quizzed me on the aspects of his speech which were most effective in reaching his audience.

On the drive home, my mind wandered to a very different time and place. I started thinking about a time in my life long before I had been diagnosed with mental illness, when I was in my early teens. I saw myself depressed and crying, because my life was not going in a direction I wanted. It was night, in the bottom half of my grandmother's townhouse, and I literally did not have a single friend. I was looking at myself in my grandmother's full-length mirror, wondering why my life had to be the way it was, and when things would ever change for me.

I curled up by that special mirror, weeping. While I leaned against the glass, lamenting my fate, I felt something startling—although it was less startling than it would have been had I not been in the middle of such sorrow.

I could hear a voice calling out to me from the mirror. "Everything is going to be alright," it said.

"Who are you?" I asked the voice.

The voice said, "I am your future self. I am happy and prosperous, and life is so much more fulfilling and happier than it is for you now.

Just endure this pain now, my son, and you will get past all of this. Things will look up for you, if you just have faith and hang in there."

I had not thought about that moment again since that time, and my mind reeled back that moment.

Now, happy and prosperous, I sent my mind back through that old mirror, as if connected to my car's rearview mirror through time and space, seeing the boy curled up on the floor, weeping because he was so unhappy with his life, and because he felt rejected by all those around him. It was as if I were really there, as I then gave comfort to that man-child, telling him how happy I was now, and how things were so much different in my present life than they were then.

What occurred next was even more startling, because I realized that I had not thought about that moment for nearly twenty years. This was the first time I had truly felt happy for an extended time. I was now thirty-three years old and had experienced so much more since I had been that young teen. But it was only at this point that it dawned on me that I was now in a position to send that message of hope to my past self.

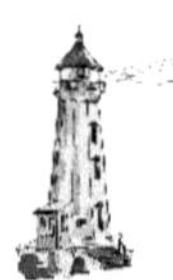

INTERESTING TIMES

After Bert had been living with us about four months, in the winter of 2007, I received good news, and it could not have come at a better time. Bert's continual insistence that he would not receive disability payments began to have a negative impact on me.

He would say, "Even if I receive benefits, it may be an entire year, before I do. I can't stay with you for a whole year. I don't want to do that to you. Why don't I just go out and get a job. Then, with that income, I can find another place to live."

I then made a decision, which in retrospect was unwise, to go along with what Bert suggested, and started helping him to look for jobs. I knew that if Bert found a job at this point in time, it would ruin any chance he would have of receiving the benefits for which he was eligible. The way the Social Security system is established, Bert would only be able to work in an extremely limited capacity after he began receiving benefits.

For two weeks, I drove Bert to a variety of locations, including the Man Power temporary work service, and to several fast food restaurants. Something contrary to all experience occurred; Bert could not seem to find a job—any job! None of the places we went to called Bert back for a job interview! He had never had a problem finding a job before in his life.

It was at that time that I received an important phone call. The manager of the Shelter Plus Program wanted to interview Bert for placement in its program! This was happy news indeed, and I felt as if I were on top of the world. Bert did not require any significant source of income while in the Shelter Plus Program, and could wait out the process for Social Security benefits, no matter how long it took, while receiving food stamps. I was willing to supply him with cigarettes and help with any necessities for as long as he needed. After being interviewed by the manager of the Shelter Plus Program, Bert was given another chance.

I drove Bert to the old apartment complex that had been such a significant part of my past, feeling a tidal wave of nostalgia crash into my psyche. These buildings had been a salvation and shelter for me when I was in direst need. I had then spent years dreaming and working to escape the place.

Now, four years later, I was thirty-three and Shelter Plus was the source of my family's salvation once again. I said hello to many of the residents. Some still remembered me and responded. Bert's apartment was on the opposite side of the building from the one in which I had lived for seven years.

Part of the agreement Bert made with the HMCMHC upon his placement in the Shelter Plus Program required him to engage in some constructive activity during the day. Bert would be attending the Adult Intensive Day Treatment Program at the HMCMHC. This was the same program that I once attended, and was parallel to the one in which I was now a psychotherapist in Decatur.

After a couple of months, Bert began to receive his disability benefits. The mental health system had come through for me once again. My faith that help is really available for people, as long as they are willing to take the appropriate steps, was renewed. The most wonderful thing was that now I was a part of the system! I helped people in situations similar to those I had experienced, both as a CMHS and as a family member of someone with SMI.

I had many factors in my favor in helping my brother get off the street. I was a social worker who knew the avenues for helping people, as well as the research available about how to work with PLMI. I could answer any of Bert's countless questions, for hours on end, about any mental health topic he could think of. I could mold Bert's understanding of mental health concepts and ways for coping with symptoms every day.

Bert was an ideal client to work with at this point. He faithfully took his medication and did not suffer a return of the psychotic symptoms that I had tried to help him cope with when I was younger. Yet we were still almost derailed by the pervasive feeling that we did not know what to expect. If Bert had been hired for one of the jobs he had applied for, his chances of receiving Social Security disability payments would have been ruined.

When I think of family members who are new to the mental health system, who have little knowledge of either the symptoms of mental illness, or the programs that are available to assist the afflicted, I want to encourage them. One component that is often missing from the lives of those first experiencing this process is hope. It is both humbling and rewarding to now be a source of hope to those people.

In 2008, Marilyn Volanino, the past president of NAMI, Decatur, and fellow Toastmaster, on hearing of my efforts to help my brother, asked me to renew my membership with NAMI. The monthly meetings and the events hosted by NAMI once again became an important part of my life, and in this way also, I felt that a piece of me that was missing was now back in place. Bert seldom participated in NAMI activities with me, preferring to remain out of the spotlight.

God is truly great, and I am thankful that he allowed me to find Bert at a time when he had reached his lowest point and was seriously ready to make a change. Bert is a part of my life that I do not intend to be distant from again. Our family was once torn apart, but now it is whole again.

My stepfather, Dave, once told me that he was familiar with a Chinese curse.

"May you live in interesting times."

I had become exceedingly accustomed to living with this curse, which had become a familiar apparition in my existence. It would have felt strange, were it not hovering about me like an old friend. I began contemplating what living in interesting times meant for me.

It occurred to me that if living in interesting times carries with it a curse, than it most assuredly carries an equally powerful and important blessing. It allowed me to see life for what it really is, to see what is essential, and to see what is superficial and fleeting. It helped me to see that the things that are important in life are not the material things, but the relationships we forge with one another. It allowed me to see that if my dreams were not rooted in higher goals then they were not worth having.

A new maxim, which is a reflection of this pearl of wisdom, formed in my mind.

"May you be blessed to live a life of interest: interest in other human beings and interest in obtaining higher goals."

When we began our journey together, I told you that when I finished describing my tale to you that I would come closer to knowing if my mind and spirit contained the makings of a great work of fiction, which I could then share with you. The conclusion I have now reached, is that there is very likely no great tale of wonder and imagination that my talents and energy will allow me to compose for you. These works have their place in helping to gain greater insight into the human condition, and they are something that will no doubt continue to inspire and feed my spirit.

I have a different purpose, however, and that is to share the events and lessons of my life with others, so that they will gain inspiration and knowledge. Whether my future life will contain additional circumstances and lessons to be shared with others remains to be seen. What is certain, though, is that I will refine my ability to communicate what wisdom I have found already, and continue to create as many lines of communication to you and to others as I can, so that they, too, can benefit from the events of my life.

I've been living in a hotel room in San Francisco for the last several days, preparing for my bicycle adventure of a lifetime. Most of my time has been spent in my room or at meetings, learning more about the 1995 Journey of Hope. I have met the other young men from around the country. They are in much better physical condition than I am and seem to know infinitely more than I do about bicycling. They go out to enjoy San Francisco's famous night life and leave me behind, since I am only twenty and can't be admitted to any of the night clubs. They've also spent a great deal of time rehearsing with the puppets with which our team is required to perform at various stops throughout our journey.

These shows are designed to foster understanding of people with disabilities in the minds of children we will meet along the way. I try to participate in the rehearsal but discover that my mind is completely unable to recall the lines I tried to memorize at home for the cloth characters. As much as I would love to breathe life into the yarn-haired dolls I am finally seeing in person, I find myself ill-equipped for the task as the lines of speech dissipate from my recollection.

On our first day of the trip we are told by our team leaders that we will participate in a bike tour of the city before actually beginning the day's journey across the Golden Gate Bridge. This scenic go round just happens to be taking place that day. I am disappointed by this since it means a lot of extra effort for my out-of-shape body to reach its first day's goal, but I'm determined to make the best of the situation.

Our team is sitting astride our bicycles in a grassy park outside San Francisco's downtown area. Hundreds of other cyclists from all over the bay area are grouped up all around us. Many of them are wearing matching uniforms. Our team's distinctive red, white, and blue cyclist uniforms set us apart from the other cyclists who aren't continuing the city bike tour across the breadth of the United States of America.

My bicycle feels strangely solid beneath me as I contemplate the many miles I have in front of me. Then we are off and pedaling, and I find myself traveling up and down the hilly streets of San Francisco. The tall buildings to either side of me make it seem that I am traveling through some sort of tunnel. Why does this all seem so familiar? Later on I will realize that I have seen these streets in the Clint Eastwood detective movies, where heavy, box-like cars are constantly chasing one another up these steep hills only to come crashing down the other side of them.

After a couple of hours in the city, we are pedaling through the green serenity of northern California trees. It won't be long until we reach the Golden Gate Bridge. The hills are just as steep to climb and the cruise down them seems far too brief an elation. What in the world have I gotten myself into?

In the years it has taken me to write my story, it has reached the early months of 2012, and many changes have taken place between then and now. Eleanor and I discovered that the many hours that it takes to write a memoir and make it available to those who would benefit from it are not conducive to a good home life when both partners work in highly stressful fields already. Wealso failed to see eye to eye on a number of important issues and found ourselves lacking in the ability to reach a successful compromise. Our marriage did not survive, and we made the mutual decision to divorce in March of 2009.

In January 2010, at the age of thirty-five, I became the President of NAMI, Decatur, serving for two years. This honor and responsibility was quite unexpected by me, and led to a variety of new experiences. I presided over monthly meetings of our members as well as quarterly board meetings. And I traveled often to Montgomery, Alabama, to represent NAMI, Decatur there. In July 2010, I traveled to Washington D.C. to represent Decatur at NAMI's national convention. I, along with NAMI representatives from across the nation, met with leaders of the United States Congress to advocate the continued provision of resources for PLMI. It was incredible to meet with family members of PLMI from all fifty states and to hear many of their stories. I also had the opportunity to meet consumers at this meeting, on a national level, who were living quite successfully in recovery from SMI.

One session that I attended at that National Conference was particularly eye opening. An older retired psychiatrist was giving a lecture in which he was discussing various aspects of schizophrenia. His plethora of knowledge about the illness focused on aspects that were not always considered by everyone in the mental health community. He described how many of the symptoms of schizophrenia are present at a young age, but they won't spike until the point at which one has their first psychotic break from reality. With women, this age tends to be in their late twenties or early thirties, and with men this age tends to be in their late teens or early twenties. In thinking back to my own childhood, I could definitely see this to be the case. Sometimes I would walk around in a kind of a trance for hours on end as my imagination ran wild. Bouts of depression and occasional paranoia were not unknown to me in these years.

Beginning in my adolescence, I was ostracized much of the time for "being different." Following one's first psychotic break with reality, after a number of years have passed, hallucinations and delusions, or positive symptoms as they are referred to, then tend to abate to some degree. He spoke about the negative symptoms that accompany schizophrenia, which include feelings of depression and lethargy. If you will recall from earlier in this work, positive symptoms are referred to as such because they add things to people that they don't want added, such as hallucinations or delusions. Negative symptoms are named thus because they take away from people things that they don't want to lose, such as energy and joy. He also spoke about the lesser known "cognitive symptoms" that are a part of the illness. Cognitive symptoms make it difficult for people to concentrate and to communicate at times. He said that these symptoms were often not given enough consideration in relation to the positive and negative symptoms, despite the fact that they too can be debilitating. As one ages these cognitive symptoms tend to worsen to a degree.

He spoke about the efficacy of the medication Clozaril and how this was considered the gold standard in terms of treating psychotic symptoms. He described how all other antipsychotic medications, including my own Seroquel were merely different variations of Clozaril. I am friends with a leader in the consumer movement who has taken Clozaril for many years and who affectionately terms the people he knows who are on this medication as the Clozaril kids. People who take Clozaril have to have blood work done on a regular basis since they are at a low risk for a condition called agranulocytosis. Because of this, it is only prescribed in cases where no other antipsychotic medication is as efficacious. While I cannot recall the name of the sage doctor gave this presentation to our small auditorium, he definitely provided me with much to consider about schizophrenia and information that I am happy to be able to share with others.

In 2010 and 2011 I also had the opportunity to present a workshop at the State Consumer Conference in Talladega, at Shocco Springs. This was the same conference that I described in some detail earlier in the book, an experience which had a profound impact upon me. I found a receptive audience there, interested in my experiences in recovery and how they could apply the lessons contained in my story to their own lives. So many of my own observations related to recovery were forged at that very site. It was truly fantastic to be able to share these with the people there.

I have also traveled all over the state as part of NAMI's, Sharing Hope program. The goal of Sharing Hope is to provide information to African American ministers, particularly in the state's Black Belt area, about ways to combat the misinformation and stigma associated with SMI. In December 2010, I left the MHCNCA to accept a position in the outpatient program at the HMCMHC. Recollections of how my own life had been saved by this very program inspired me to continue my work as a helping professional there. I also began serving as the president of Our Place, CRDC. In 2012, immediately prior to publication of this work, I won the RESPECT Award, the recipients of which are chosen by consumers across the state of Alabama for their contributions to PLMI.

Whenever I am asked if it is worth it to sacrifice my time in an effort to fight mental illness and improve the lives of others, my answer is always the same: "Yes."

We have reached the end of the journey at a fine hotel in Charleston, South Carolina. I have seen Fort Sumter, the starting point of the American Civil War, from across the water, and find that it holds my attention for a surprisingly short span of time. It is longer though than seeing Alcatraz island at the beginning of the trip in San Francisco, which I don't remember seeing at all. I am dressed in a suit for the closing ceremony of the 1995 Journey of Hope. My entire appearance has changed since the beginning of my journey, and I am now the very picture of physical fitness. In the hallway of the hotel, one of my buddies from the trip tells me, "Wow, Jim, you really do look like a lawyer in your suit." I smile at these words of encouragement as we make our way to the elevator and then down into a darkened ballroom.

We line up to hear who has won the leadership award for our trip. He is the man who broke his collarbone, after crashing into a car. We all clap for him, reflecting on the irony that we would have all likely picked this likeable man for the award, even if he hadn't been injured. We all see him as the most positive member of the team.

I receive no award, but we all hear our names called aloud to signify our completion of this event. After my name is called I hear a remarkable thing: the team members all seem to be clapping and cheering for me louder than they did anyone else! The applause continues for an interminable length of time before it finally dissipates into silence. I did not expect this outpouring of emotion connected to the calling of my name. It seems to me as if the team members doing the cheering didn't expect it either. I can't stop wondering why in the world that just happened.

TWENTY-FIVE-TWENTY-FIVE

The new year of 2021 is fresh as I work on revising *The Mindful Son.* The Covid-19 pandemic is raging, though the new vaccine offers a ray of hope for all. In the eight and a half intervening years since I first published, I have experienced much. I continue to work as an outpatient therapist for a community MHC but now my post is in the small town of Cullman, Alabama. I have grown in my level of experience, which has only added to my level of effectiveness as a clinician.

Following the first publication of the book, I was asked to speak at a number of venues, one of which was at my Alma Matter, the University of Alabama where I spoke to a group of 250 students. Incidentally, I also spoke in Auburn, Alabama, the town which hosts UA's rival school Auburn University, but for the MHC there. The setting for this speech was in a Methodist church with beautiful stained-glass windows. Speaking in a church setting always seems to give me an extra spark of inspiration. I am a member of University Baptist Church in Huntsville and participate primarily online due to geography and the need for social distancing.

A big change for college campuses has been the advent of NAMI on Campus, where students experiencing mental illness can meet and interact with other students with many of the same issues. This would have been of enormous value to me when I was a student trying to finish up my own degree, and I am thankful this source of support is now available to the next generation of consumers.

Another improvement in the lives of many consumers has been the advent of long-lasting injectables of the newer antipsychotic medications. Earlier in my recovery story, I was injected with one of the older antipsychotic medications called Prolixin and suffered terrible side-effects for a time as a result. Years after that, around the time, I first started practicing as a therapist, in 2004, injectable versions of some of the newer antipsychotic medications became available, which treat both positive and negative symptoms being sold by the ever-present pharmaceutical representatives who visited the MHC. At that time, these medications were very expensive and not in use to a great extent in public mental health. Over the years, however, these medications have become more affordable and are now in much greater use. I have had the chance to see remarkable results with people on these medications in many instances and would encourage people to consider this option if oral medications are not having the desired effect. With injectables, one only has to remember to take them either once per two weeks, once per month, or even once per three months, as opposed to every single day. It also removes a number of non-compliance considerations from the table. While certainly not for everyone with psychotic, or in some cases, manic symptoms, they are definitely a convenience and benefit to many. I spoke to groups of mental health professionals who said they also saw benefits of these medications for the consumers they worked with.

The speeches that I was invited to give focused heavily on ways to overcome obstacles. I would provide my audience with a list of the ten tenets that had guided me down my path to recovery. These were on decorative paper resembling an unfurled scroll to emphasize their importance. These ten tenets are as follows:

1. Always surround yourself with positive people who believe in you.
2. Good things often happen in their own time.
3. Persistent and unfailing effort is the key to accomplishing your goals.
4. Don't feel down on yourself if you haven't accomplished all of your goals yet.
5. Achieving one goal will propel you toward the next one.
6. Never forget the power of miracles and acknowledge them when they occur.
7. Avoid intoxicating substances as well as toxic relationships.

8. Take time out to recharge your battery and do some things that you enjoy.
9. Every decision that we make is a calculated risk.
10. Recognize the opportunities that come your way and go for it!

In my speeches, I would elaborate on the meaning of these principles in greater detail to my audience, using examples from my recovery story to illustrate their power in action. My audience seemed to benefit from these speeches and often offered positive feedback.

In 2013, I travelled to the NAMI National Convention in San Antonio, where my book was on sale at the bookstore along with other publications related to mental health. While there, I walked along the famous River Walk, which I'd only seen before watching the NBA finals when the San Antonio Spurs basketball team was playing in them. Spurs merchandise could be seen just about everywhere someone traveled there. I found some relief from the intense July Summer sun at the Alamo and the gorgeous botanical garden which was planted just behind it.

One of the speakers at this conference was Dr. Xavier Amadore, author of the book, I Am Not Sick, I Don't Need Help: How to Help Someone with Mental Illness Accept Treatment. This book was inspired by his efforts at helping his brother Henry, to accept treatment for schizophrenia. I later read this book and found it to be quite insightful. In his speech, he described his family's story as well as concepts from the book including the condition known as anosognosia.

According to NAMI, anosognosia is a symptom that affects about thirty percent of people with schizophrenia and twenty percent of people with bipolar disorder. It is an extreme inability for someone to accurately perceive their own self-image as having a mental illness, despite clear evidence to the contrary. Anosognosia comes from the Greek meaning "to not know a disease"

It's important for family members and mental health providers to be aware that people with this serious medical condition are not just being stubborn or trying to be uncooperative with treatment when they don't want care. They genuinely don't believe they have the illness and don't want to take medication for a condition they don't believe impacts them. To demonstrate this concept, Dr. Amadore pulled a random lady out of the audience and asked her if she had diabetes. She said "no" and he then proceeded to try and convince her that she did in fact have diabetes. The intentionally awkward exchange illustrated the concept of anosognosia perfectly. He went on to talk about how the best treatment approach for some people with this condition is to help them see the benefits of receiving care even though they did not actually believe they had a mental illness. Remaining out of the hospital is one such motivator.

Some news publications took an interest in my own story, including the Huffington Post, who featured a related article. I also did some interviews for radio and television. Mike Autrey, the Director of the Office of Consumer Relations for the state of Alabama took an interest in my story, and two articles in the state's consumer magazine, Listen, were published about it.

Mike also invited me to serve on a number of boards for the state and to earn my certification as a Peer Support Specialist. In 2015, I served as the treasurer for the Alabama Peer Support Specialist Association, as well as on the state's Advocacy Advisory Board. The beginning of 2015 also marks the last time I smoked a cigarette, and I'm thankful to say that I have been nicotine free ever since.

In 2016, I left Alabama to work for the Veteran's Administration in Central Illinois as a

social worker for their inpatient unit for two years. The lessons that I learned there are invaluable and remain an important part of my practice today.

Bert is presently living in a group home in Athens, Alabama and is in the process of moving into a more independent setting as soon as he can. He has now graduated from using a cell phone to using a smart phone, which I was able to painstakingly teach him how to utilize. Our relationship remains close.

When I first move to Danville, Illinois, a small town twenty miles west of Indiana, my landlord drives me to a hanger that houses some World War II fighter planes. He knows that I have an interest in them because I told him about my grandfatherly cousin who flew them in that war. "They are a lot bigger than I had imagined, for some reason." I tell him. While in Washington D.C. six years prior to that I had visited the Air and Space Museum there, which had many similarities to the Air and Space Museum of my own hometown of Huntsville. I spend most of my time during that trip with Reverend Thomas and his family, who are African American, and who are part of the NAMI Sharing Hope program, which provides information about mental health to primarily African American ministers. His wife is a long-time social worker for NARH, though I never met her there when I was a patient, and their son Eli is sixteen and playing football in high school. We leave the Air and Space Museum, watching horse drawn buggies carrying tourists down the street, and make our way to the newly built Native American Museum.

At the National Mall, we pass by the National Christmas Tree and read the plaque that says that it had been there since 1974. We have no knowledge that the next year it will be blasted to cinders by lightening. Reverend Thomas will also contract cancer and pass away around that time, leaving a hole in all of the hearts of the people that knew him.

We see the Washington Monument in the distance and are impressed by it, but don't get a chance to see it up close. "Most people don't realize that the tip of it is made of aluminum." I remark. We also get a good glimpse of the World War II Memorial, but again don't have a chance to really see it up close.

We stop at the Women's Vietnam Memorial for a moment while Reverend Thomas collects his thoughts. "The larger Vietnam Memorial is just over there. I'd like to see that too!" I said.

"I don't think I can handle that right now," he said, head lowered.

I realized that he probably had close friends that died in Vietnam and would be overwrought with feelings of grief if we did. "I'll surely get a chance to see it another time," I said to myself.

We see the Lincoln Monument up ahead and make our way there. Up, up, the giant white marble steps we go. The sheer sense of enormity of it all is staggering. At the top of the steps, we see Abraham Lincoln in gargantuan form, reclining on his huge marble throne in blue shadow. The walls of the monument are inscribed with enormous lines of the speeches he wrote. We feel overwhelmed by the scale of everything there, and clearly none of us has seen anything like this before. We head back down the steep, crowded steps snapping photos of each other many times along the way.

...Back in Danville, Illinois in 2018, I'm touring the local War Museum with my brother Bert, who is in town for a visit. Surrounded by endless rows of uniforms, weapons, and medals we can't help but recall our stepfather, Dave's home, which was filled with model planes, tanks, and even a large zeppelin that he had glued together and painted by hand. His home also housed rifles from all time periods that he had refurbished himself. The steel helmets and brimmed officer's hats with gold leaf that we see displayed in the museum were like the ones back home that we'd tried on ourselves a hundred times before. Dave's home town of Indianapolis, Indiana is only an hour away. Ironically, I had also visited Indianapolis five years before I moved up north in order to see the Indy 500 auto race with my friend, Tommy. If you will recall, Tommy had helped talk me out of suicide much earlier on in my recovery. Even more ironically, his parents were actually from the Illiana community that VA Illiana was named for, where I ended up working for the Veteran's Administration. Illiana is a combination of the names of the states Illinois and Indiana, since the VA there was located very near the border of the two states. After the race Tommy, and I grilled hamburgers in the field where we had parked before the race, while contemplating all we had seen that day. It was the 100th anniversary of the race that year, and someone had constructed a monstrous Hot Wheels track with giant loops to drive life sized cars through. Jim Neighbors, the man who starred in Gomer Pile, and Florence Henderson, the mother of The Brady Bunch, sang songs before the race, as was the annual tradition. Back in our hotel room, I'm able to watch a replay of the race which allows me to piece together what the noisy whizzing blurs I had witnessed actually did that day. The winner of the race that year, Dan Wheldon, is Australian, and will die in a car wreck at race a couple of years later. When Bert and I go to Indianapolis together we don't go to the race, but instead we spend time in the arcade and restaurant known as Dave and Buster's.

Our stepfather, Dave's Alma Matter, Purdue University in West Lafayette, Indiana is one hour away as well, and I've visited it a number of times while living in the area. One of the routes from Danville to West Lafayette allows you to see mile upon mile of giant white windmills with three thin blades rotating in the wind.

Back in my small apartment in Danville, Illinois, Bert is wearing a mood ring that he purchased from his winnings at Dave and Buster's. Its slowly shifting colors seem to capture and hold his attention for a long stretch of time.

It's now 2010, and I'm with a group of fellow PLMI for a mental health field trip at a Native American festival taking place around giant mounds of earth that were once used for religious rites in a town called Oakville in Alabama. A giant staircase ascends to the top of one of the mounds which is flat on top. The other, smaller mound is covered in trees, and no one is allowed to walk there. A large pond lies near the Indian mounds and was likely dug by hand to supply the earth for the mounds. On this day there is an annual festival celebrating Native American culture taking place so the entire area is crowded with children of all ages. Traversing the long bridge that crosses the deep blue water of the pond is cumbersome, as a result.

There are vendors there who sell hand-crafted items. I purchase a large turkey feather fan and some sage to burn and then waft upon myself for ritual cleansing. A pow wow dance is happening there as well. I think back to a past pow wow I attended in Tuscaloosa while I was living with Kim and finishing up my bachelor's degree at UA in 1997. The same funnel cakes covered with powdered sugar which were on sale there are available at this pow wow as well. Tuscaloosa lies near another smaller town called Moundville. It is also the home to some large Native American mounds. I have never visited the actual Mounds in Moundville, but I will visit the town on two occasions in my future. The first occasion is 2012, when I have been asked to share my recovery story to a group of black ministers congregating at the AME church there to learn more about mental health issues. The other occasion is when I'm traveling by car to see the UA play in the Sugar Bowl in New Orleans in 2019. I'm riding there with my friend Tim and we make a stop in Moundville to visit Tim's niece. The UA goes on to win that game and then the National Championship Game after that against The University of Georgia, in one of the most dramatic endings seen in college sports history. These two games will be juxtaposed in my mind such that it feels as if I was actually in person for the national championship game and not just the Sugar Bowl. The nation's largest

Native American mound, Cahokia, is in Illinois, but I don't have a chance to visit it in person either.

Back in 2010, at the festival in Oakville, a loud cannon booms out a shocking wave of sound like thunder about every fifteen minutes or so. There is a booth that showcases blacksmithing from the nineteenth century near where the cannon lies. Two months after that festival I will visit the Native American Museum in Washinton D.C. I will see rows of sabers exhibited at the Native American museum there. Winchester rifles will also be on display. Reverend Thomas will point to a placard that describes the curse that the Winchester family supposedly had cast upon them because of the number of people who died from that rifle. For now, in Oakville, though, my mind drifts back to a time when I'm out west with the Journey of Hope. A couple of my fellow riders and I walk into a rocky enclave enclosed by cold stone which was once utilized by Native Americans for ceremonial purposes. Inside we stare in awe at a naturally cut stone chair that looks very much like a throne. In what state in the country this was in or if any one of us chose to sit in it ourselves I cannot, for the life of me, recall. Warping ahead in time to 2021, a prequel for The Mindful Son begins to crystalize and take form in my mind. The future remains a beautiful mystery.

SPREAD THE WORD.

The Mindful Son: A Beacon of Hope Through the Storm of Mental Illness is now available through Alpha Centauri Press.

To find out more about ordering the book or to access recorded interviews with James or related articles, visit www.jameshickman-themindfulson.weebly.com.

To contact James about speaking to your organization, email him at JamesHickman9242@gmail.com or contact him by phone at 256-323-9005.

ABOUT THE AUTHOR

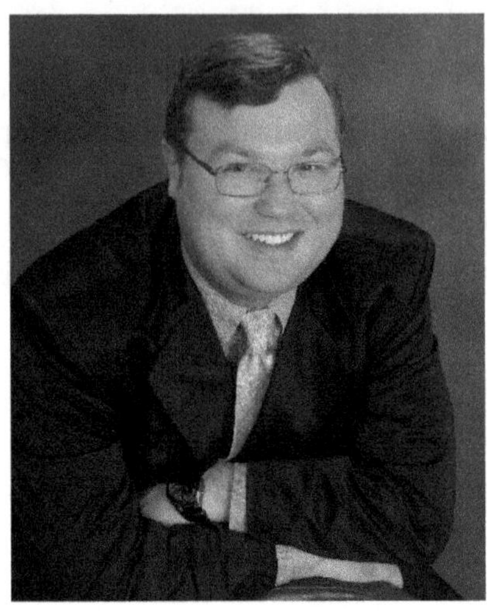

James Hickman is a Licensed Certified Social Worker in the state of Alabama and works as a mental health therapist for WellStone. He is also a Certified Peer Support Specialist in Alabama and has served as the Treasurer for the Alabama Peer Support Specialist Association. James has served as the President of The National Alliance on Mental Illness in Decatur.

He is a Co-Founder of Our Place, a consumer-run drop-in center in Huntsville. James has served on the Board of Directors of Wings Across Alabama, the primary voice for consumers of mental health services throughout the state. He has also served on the Advisory Board of the Alabama Disability Advocacy Program, the Consumer Advisory Board to the Associate Commissioner of Mental Health in Alabama, and the Advisory Board of NAMI's Sharing Hope, a program designed to share information about mental health with ministers primarily in the Black Belt area. James received the Beacon of Hope award from the Huntsville/Madison County Mental Health Center in 2007 and the RESPECT award from his fellow consumers across the state of Alabama in 2012. He has had the privilege of speaking to a wide array of audiences about overcoming obstacles to quality mental health.

PRAISE FOR THE MINDFUL SON

"James' book takes the reader through the roller coaster life of mental illness. Anyone who suffers from mental illness or has a family member or friend who suffers from mental illness will find comfort in this remarkable journey."

James Walsh, Ex-Officio, Executive Committee National
Alliance on Mental Illness, Alabama

"The Mindful Son offers hope-while the challenges that Hickman encounters are tremendous and, at times seem overwhelming, his story illuminates the possibility of recovery. For anyone whose life is touched by mental illness, this book offers valuable insight."

David Hitt, author of *Homesteading Space: The Skylab Story* and *Bold they Rise: The Space Shuttle Early Years, 1972-1986*

"This is a book that should be read by everyone involved in the treatment of persons with schizophrenia, including family, psychiatrists, advocates, and therapists. James' story is brimming with hope. I am proud to be working with him as a colleague at the mental health center."

Dr. Bill Goodson, psychiatrist, author, and one of the
founders of the Huntsville-Madison County
Mental Health Center.

"Jim's story of courage, perseverance and determination is an inspiration. His is a story, not of dealing with his personal struggles with mental illness but rather a story of success, hope and recovery. I recommend it to anyone whose life has been touched by adversity."

Mike Autrey, Director
Alabama Office of Consumer Relations

"Hickman looks at the world of mental health through a prism of unique experience."

Robert Hermes, Director
Wings Across Alabama

www.ingramcontent.com/pod-product-compliance
Lightning Source LLC
Chambersburg PA
CBHW071405090426
42737CB00011B/1365

* 9 7 8 0 9 8 5 0 8 5 6 3 6 *